Y0-CCN-438

Effective Approaches
to Patients' Behavior

GLADYS B. LIPKIN, R.N., M.S., is certified by the American Nurses' Association as a generalist and specialist in psychiatric and mental health nursing, and by the ANA and the Nurses' Association of the American College of Obstetrics and Gynecology in maternal and neonatal nursing. In addition to her independent practice as a nurse psychotherapist in Bayside, New York, Ms. Lipkin is a clinical nurse specialist, lecturer, and prepared childbirth (Lamaze) instructor.

ROBERTA G. COHEN, R.N., M.S., is nurse psychotherapist and clinical specialist at Mercy Hospital, Rockville Centre, New York. An independent nurse psychotherapist in private practice in North Merrick, New York, she is also a lecturer and an adjunct assistant clinical professor in the department of nursing at Adelphi University.

Effective Approaches
to Patients' Behavior

Second Edition

Gladys B. Lipkin, R.N., M.S.
Roberta G. Cohen, R.N., M.S.

SPRINGER PUBLISHING COMPANY
New York

Springer Publishing Company, Inc.
200 Park Avenue South
New York, N.Y. 10003

First edition, 1973
80 81 82 83 84 / 10 9 8 7 6 5 4 3 2 1

Library of Congress Cataloging in Publication Data

Lipkin, Gladys B
    Effective approaches to patients' behavior.

    Bibliography: p. 259–71
    Includes index.
    1. Nurse and patient. 2. Sick—Psychology.
I. Cohen, Roberta G., joint author. II. Title.
RT86.L56   1980   610.73'.069   79-23046
ISBN 0-8261-1491-1
ISBN 0-8261-1492-x pbk.

Printed in the United States of America

When two nurses who have busy and full lives decide to coauthor a book, they have to count on the highest degree of understanding and cooperation from those they love. We were fortunate to have had the support and encouragement of our husbands, Drs. Murray Cohen and Nathan Lipkin, of our children, Anne and David Cohen, and Rebecca, Alan, and Harriet Lipkin, and of our parents. Although we have thanked them privately, we want also to do so publicly.

Contents

Preface

Forty percent of all hospital beds in the United States are now occupied by psychiatric patients. Statistically, this represents a 10 percent decrease in the hospital load over the past few years. However, this does not mean that the number of patients under care has dropped. In fact, more are now receiving care, but in nontraditional (and often inadequate) settings. Hospitalization is often sought in crisis situations, with the result that emotional problems do not manifest themselves solely in patients in psychiatric units. Health workers in the community and in the general hospital, as well as those in psychiatric institutions, are often confronted by patients with symptoms of emotional disturbances which do not require treatment by a psychiatrist, yet are serious enough to require meaningful and assertive intervention on the worker's part. Health workers may shy away from such patients because they are not certain of what to say, how to say it, or when to initiate the approach to the patient. Often they fear that their actions may cause further deterioration in the patient's emotional or somatic state.

The purpose of this book is to present the problem areas in which workers frequently become involved, and which necessitate on-the-spot action. The worker who is familiar with behavior patterns and the do's and don'ts of intervention will be able to function in this role with ease, understanding, and effectiveness. At the same time, the worker's action gives the patient an opportunity to learn how to cope with immediate stresses. Emotional growth is also fostered through these interactions.

As nurse psychotherapists, both authors have worked extensively with patients who present difficulties manifested by changes in their emotional and/or physical states, and with the staffs who care for these patients. Our experiences have reinforced our belief that the worker who is acquainted with basic psychiatric techniques and concepts is able to approach his patients confidently and, hopefully, successfully.

As stated in the first edition, we both feel the need for a short manual that describes problem behavior, offers a discussion of the dynamics involved, and suggests approaches to be used with the patient. With this second edition of our book we again hope to create a practical, concise, and informative guide for all health workers involved in the care of patients who demonstrate some aspect of emotional disturbance, whether they be in the community, in the general hospital, or in a psychiatric setting. For this edition, we have added several chapters and expanded the previous material in order to clarify ideas or present additional concepts which we have found useful.

We have incorporated material from our own experiences in the attempt to increase the reader's understanding of various personality and behavior disturbances. The section on the interview and crisis intervention includes information intended to help health workers acquire or improve their skills in communicating with the patient. Although we recognize that professional competence can be developed only through actual clinical practice, we hope the use of this book will expedite its acquisition.

Our goals will have been met if we give our readers a sense of *what* to do and *how* to do it, along with some comprehension of *why* we have found particular approaches to be helpful.

May, 1979

GLADYS B. LIPKIN
ROBERTA G. COHEN

Acknowledgments

Many coworkers, teachers, and friends, coming from a variety of disciplines, have helped me focus on the needs of patients and health workers. I am personally grateful to all of them, as well as to my many patients, who have shared experiences that stimulated the writing of this edition. Again, this book would not be possible without the assistance of our typist, Mrs. Valerie Koneski, and the helpful staff at Springer Publishing Company.

GBL

Since the first edition of this book was published, continued opportunity has been given to me to grow personally and professionally as a clinical nurse specialist and nurse psychotherapist at Mercy Hospital. I am grateful to Dr. Gerald F. Perry, Medical Director, and Dr. Brian F. Fitzsimmons, Administrative Director, Department of Psychiatry, Mercy Hospital, for their understanding and support of my work. Additionally, I wish to thank the entire staff in the Department of Psychiatry, Mercy Hospital, for their friendship and the sharing of so many happy work years with me.

RGC

PART ONE

Overview of Interpersonal Relations and Preventive Psychiatry

Looking at the Patient

The doctor leaves the room, and one patient begins to shriek and cry at what he has told her. Her fears have been justified . . . her illness is very serious. In the next bed, her roommate lies composed and silent. Nurses run to the shouting patient, and try to calm and soothe her. They take no notice of her neighbor.

Actually, each patient has just been given the same unhappy diagnosis by the doctor. Perhaps their differing reactions are due in part to differences in their backgrounds. Each may be imitating her own forebears and the methods they used in handling personal troubles. Both are upset, angry, and anxious, but their ways of showing these feelings obviously differ. If we assess only the reaction without viewing it in the light of the patient's background, we may think of a noisy reaction as unnecessary and disturbing to other patients as well as ourselves. On the other hand, we may misjudge the depth of the quiet person's feelings simply because she is so quiet. In truth, the second patient may be in greater need of comforting, for she has a much more limited outlet for her feelings and worries.

Determining whether the behavior of a patient is "normal" must include an evaluation of the circumstances in which that behavior takes place. For example, the person who wears a bathing suit to a barbecue held at a swimming area would be viewed as acting properly. However, if the same person wore a bathing suit to a formal dinner, he would certainly be looked at askance.

The patient's background is largely responsible for his daily actions and reactions while he is in the hospital. If hot water has been hard to come by throughout his life, and baths have been once-a-week affairs, the nurse is unlikely to be able to convince him that he really needs a full bed bath every day, unless she does some effective health teaching. If breakfast has always been bypassed, and between-meal snacks are a family habit, he will probably follow the same pattern in the hospital unless he can be made to realize that regular, well-balanced meals are a more healthful way of satisfying his hunger. Reviewing the patient's background will help the nurse to understand that his behavior is not based on a desire to be dirty, and that he does not really want to be difficult at mealtime. However, there is a good chance that he may change his ingrained pattern of behavior if he can be convinced that other patterns are better for him. In any event, once the staff becomes conscious of his life style, it is improbable that they will continue to think of him as "that dirty old man who gives us so much trouble at mealtime."

The cultural factors that have shaped the sick person's behavior in the past will continue to affect his actions wherever he may be now. In some cultures, the sick or elderly have been traditionally cared for at home, and hospitals have been considered places only for the dying. The patient who is part of such a culture may feel abandoned when he is removed from his family and taken to the hospital for some minor procedure. In other cultures, the display of emotions is approved, so the patient may enjoy crying. In still other groups stoicism is encouraged, and the individual learns to maintain complete control—at least superficially. Discovering these background factors helps to improve understanding and leads to more meaningful relations between patients and the hospital staff.

Religious practices account for certain behavior patterns exhibited by some patients. The Catholic who refuses to go to surgery before receiving communion is not being uncooperative. Neither is the orthodox Jew who refuses to eat non-kosher food. The Jehovah's Witness who vehemently refuses a blood transfusion places his religious tenets above immediate health considerations. Should those with differing religious beliefs refuse to honor the convictions of such patients? Should we be furious that the operating room schedule is delayed, that the kitchen must make special dietary arrangements, or that the need for blood must be reconsidered? Do we have the right to add to the patient's discomfort by being angry and argumentative while trying to convince him to do what we want him to do? Showing respect for the religious beliefs of others, no matter how widely they vary from our own, helps one to make an honest assessment of the patient's behavior. He certainly is neither stubborn nor uncooperative if he tries, even in a time of stress, to adhere to the teachings of a lifetime.

The patient from a low socioeconomic group may view his placement in a single room as a luxury. He may not want to "bother" the staff, and therefore gets out of bed to go to the bathroom even when on strict bed rest. At the other end of the scale, the patient from a high socioeconomic group may complain that the paint is chipped off the bed, or that the linen is not changed often enough. He may demand a great deal from the staff, even though he is permitted to be up and around ad libitum. Either patient may be thought of as a "problem" unless viewed in the context of his background. Acknowledgment by the staff of the first patient's need to be completely independent, and of the second one's need for a coterie of people to order about will help both patients understand their own behavior. Often, such a simple phrase as, "It must be difficult for you to have to depend on others for all your needs," or "It must be frustrating for you not to have people available to help you immediately," will enable the patient to think through his reaction to his present situation.

Often when a member of one of the medical disciplines becomes a patient he presents many problems to the hospital staff. He tries to guess his diagnosis from tests being done. He may question the necessity or wisdom of medications or treatments ordered for him. He often will not ask questions about himself directly, but rather will say, "This test is usually done for cancer, isn't it?" He interprets an evasive answer as an indication that he does indeed have cancer. In such an instance, it may be helpful for the nurse to say, "Yes, it may be done for cancer, but it is also used to confirm other diagnoses as well. Your doctor will tell you about the other conditions that he was considering when he ordered the test."

The health professional who has been involved with patients in the clinical situation may become anxious when methods other than those he is familiar with are used to carry out procedures. He may note that sterile equipment appears to have become contaminated, or that he would do things differently. If the staff can discuss these differences with him and offer a theoretical basis for the techniques being used, he will probably feel more at ease. His knowledge and experience may be broader than that of many of the staff. For example, if he is the medical director of the service staff, members may have to remind themselves that being a patient is as difficult for him as caring for him is for the staff. All his expertise will not make him less anxious than any other patient. Perhaps, knowing as much as he does may *increase* his anxiety. Air in the intravenous tubing, crooked needles, contaminated equipment all add to his stress, particularly as he tries to have the situation corrected without showing his distrust of the staff. His desire to be a "good" patient may increase his anxiety even further as he tries to reassure himself that others can be knowledgeable as he is, and that his care will be as excellent as any that he would provide for one of his own patients. Considering these factors, it is not difficult to understand why he questions everyone and everything.

Nonprofessional hospital volunteers or their family members who are hospitalized frequently present problems in that they often have preconceived notions of what their care should include. They may misunderstand procedures or test results, but be unwilling to admit their lack of knowledge by asking questions. In addition, they may request special privileges because of their association with the hospital. They expect an acknowledgment of their services, and may be upset if staff members do not recognize them as very important people.

Previous hospital experiences also modify patients' behavior. If this is yet another admission for the same condition, the patient may be very upset and discouraged, for it indicates that he is not improving. The patient with heart or kidney disease, or with diabetes, may feel that following the rigid limitations of diet does not make a difference, that he will be sick whether he follows or disregards the rules. He may be angry that he has deprived himself of foods that are forbidden but enjoyable, only to become ill anyway. Talking about his feelings will help, because it gives him the chance to ventilate his anger as well as find out where he may have made mistakes. (Patients on a salt restricted diet have been known to scrupulously avoid sodium chloride while freely using monosodium glutamate, not realizing that the sodium is the harmful substance.) The approach might be, "How do you feel about being back in the hospital?

Some people find it frustrating to stay on an unappealing diet and still become ill. Let's take a look at your food intake and see if you might have overlooked something that is responsible for your present difficulty."

The patient's previous hospital experiences may have involved the illness of family members or friends rather than himself. He may remember these incidents pleasantly or apprehensively, depending on the quality of the care they received and the outcome of the hospitalization. If a biopsy was performed, and a negative report received, he remembers the hospital as a happy place. If, on the other hand, the report was positive, and the friend or relative later died, his memories of the hospital may be very distressing ones. When the patient is relatively well and comfortable, visitors tend not to notice hospital shortcomings. This is particularly true if staff members have been helpful to the patient. On the other hand, staff members who may be short-tempered or argumentative often cause visitors (as well as patients) to become hostile and angry. The individual who enters a hospital after being involved in a pleasant or unpleasant previous experience, whether his own or someone else's, will have initial feelings that are colored by that experience.

Children are particularly influenced by how they were cared for during prior hospitalizations. They remember the attitudes of staff members in great detail, especially in relation to truthfulness. If a child had been told that a procedure would be painless, and found the opposite to be true, he now anticipates that every procedure will be painful. Conversely, he will place greater trust in the staff if, on a previous hospitalization, he was told before a procedure was to be done, exactly what to expect. Being in the hospital is less frightening and less anxiety-provoking when the child knows that health workers are reliable, supportive people who do not enjoy causing pain, but are truthful about it when it is unavoidable. Memories of unhappy childhood hospitalizations continue to haunt some patients through the years and resistance to later admissions may be based on those memories.

Some patients who are admitted to either a general or a psychiatric hospital have a long-standing history of abnormal behavior for which they have not been previously hospitalized, either because the symptoms were not severe enough, or because the family insisted upon keeping the patient at home. Some of these patients have created an unreal world to which they retreat so as to protect themselves against any feelings of anxiety produced by the real world that surrounds them. Their actions may be subject to orders from some invisible power in that secret world, their vision may be distorted, and their language may become unintelligible due to this power. The unreal world is, in a sense, the patient's protection against the unbearable feelings that he is experiencing in the real world. Some patients move back and forth between their two worlds, resorting to the unreal one only at times of great personal stress, and then they seem unable to see, hear, or feel anything going on around them.

Ujhely writes of *"sustaining the patient through the experience,"*[1] an important concept in meeting the needs of *all* patients, but especially of those who lose contact with reality. Using this concept, the health worker must first become aware of the patient's *perception* of the current situation. How does what is happening appear to the patient? His perceptions may differ from those of others in similar situations because of his physical state (as when he has severe or constant pain), the culture in which he has lived (as the Amish farmer who regards the taking of x-rays as against the dictum of having "graven images"), or his accumulated knowledge.

The second factor the worker needs to be aware of is the patient's *interpretation* of what is happening. He may be distorting what he has perceived because of his extreme anxiety, or inability to think things through properly (as the patient who refuses to have her chest shaved for a breast biopsy "because it will make hair grow on my chest later").

A third factor for the worker to note is the patient's *response,* which will depend on his capacity to cope with a given situation in light of his ability, his background, and his previously learned responses in similar situations.

Having assessed the patient's perception, interpretation, and response, the worker can then move on to *sustain* the patient. This is an all-encompassing term that indicates ways in which the patient may be helped to cope with the situation now at hand. It calls for sensitivity on the part of the worker, the ability to let the patient's experience take precedence

1. G. Ujhely. *Determinants of the Nurse-Patient Relationship.* New York: Springer Publishing Company, Inc., 1968, p. 93.

over the niceties of hospital care, accepting the patient even when he is in his unreal world, and not forcing other standards of behavior upon him until he is ready for change. It may take a long time before the patient feels safe enough to change. This will usually happen as a result of his trusting those who care for him in ways that indicate sincere concern for him as a human being.

Travelbee[2] notes the distorted perception of both the givers and receivers of care when the term "patient" is used. The individual may easily be dehumanized when he is stereotyped and categorized according to his particular illness. Such thinking dulls the ability of the health worker to regard the patient as a person with unique qualifications, one who must be regarded in terms of his background (ethnic, cultural, socioeconomic, etc.), physical status, home environment, and current problems.

The health worker can be of greatest help to those in his care when he is empathic and sympathetic, but not immobilized by either of these reactions. Patients sense that the worker understands them and wants to help. For some patients, the worker is the only individual in the world to whom they can tell all their worries, sorrows, and expectations. Their close emotional involvement with family members and friends may make such disclosures too painful. Hopefully, the worker is able to tolerate what is being said, and does not turn a confiding patient off with such trite phrases as "Don't worry," "Everything will be all right," "Your family still loves you." If the worker becomes involved (but not incapacitated by that involvement), he can not only help the patient through his experience of illness, but can also help him learn how to deal with life more meaningfully when healthy.

Almost always, patients fear a hospital experience. They fear such unknown factors as the diagnosis, the treatment, the outcome, and the type of care they will receive. Some will conceal their feelings with a veneer of humor or boredom. Others will cling to hospital personnel, much as children do, seeking scraps of information about themselves. Occasionally patients will cry, a most upsetting spectacle for some health workers,

2. J. Travelbee. *Interpersonal Aspects of Nursing.* 2nd ed. Philadelphia: F. A. Davis Company, 1971, pp. 36–38.

who communicate their feeling by what they say and do. The pat answer, "There, there, don't cry," neither stops the crying nor helps the patient. Telling him to "pull yourself together" makes him feel that he is regarded as inadequate and that the worker is looking down upon him. The patient needs to feel the strength and empathy of a worker who can stay with him, one who is not upset by the tears. Verbal communication helps to make the patient feel less guilty about his tears. "I realize how upset you are. Sometimes tears ease that feeling," implies that the worker believes the patient can mobilize untapped strengths within himself. This encourages his belief that the worker recognizes him as a person with assets still to be used. The feeling that someone else believes in him often furnishes the motivating force for the patient to find those strengths. Nonverbal communication is equally important. An arm around the patient's shoulder, a hand on his arm, or a gentle hand helping to wipe away the tears all indicate to the patient that there is acceptance of what might ordinarily be unacceptable. He can still retain his dignity, knowing that he is looked upon as a very human being.

Looking at the Health Worker

The health worker's observation and understanding of the patient is a prime consideration in determining the care that is to be given. But unless the worker understands himself, his perceptions of the patient may be incorrect. The worker, as well as the patient, brings to the bedside a value system that is based on socioeconomic, cultural, health, religious, educational, and work backgrounds. It is impossible for a worker to make an insightful evaluation of the patient if he considers his own standards impeccable and uses them as the basis for evaluating the patient. Even though the professional's standards may be "perfect" within his own social group, he cannot expect to develop therapeutic relationships by applying his beliefs indiscriminately when evaluating the status and needs of patients.

The worker usually enters one of the health professions for special reasons. For many, the chance to help others is the prime consideration. For others, the stimulus may be provided by the availability and stability of job opportunities, the status of belonging to a respected profession, or even the prodding of parents, relatives, and teachers. Some are influenced by serious illnesses they have had as children, or books they have read about heroic medical achievements. And there are also those who can give no conscious reason for having chosen a career in one of the health services.

The health worker who has led a sheltered life, protected by environment and parents, may find it difficult to become attuned to the needs of others. On the other hand, the worker whose life had been full of problems, and who has not had his own needs met, may find it equally difficult to hear a cry for help. It is not that these workers are unwilling to be

11

helpful. Rather, they are unable to assess situations because their backgrounds are limited in scope and experience. Neither worker has had the opportunity to compare his own background with that of others; thus, neither one understands how different rearing might have provided him with greater insight and empathy in his relationships with patients.

The worker who was reared in a home in which family members always subdued their emotions may be uncomfortable when faced with a highly charged situation. It is easier to become busy with other tasks than to face the obvious difficulty of entering a patient's room when anticipating a tirade. The patient who cries, moans, screams at relatives and staff is looked upon as an unpleasant individual, one to be avoided if at all possible. The worker may see no reason to accept abuse, particularly if he himself has always been a kindly, "good" person, respected by others. He regards the patient as nasty and ungrateful, and does not think in terms of understanding the patient's umet needs.

The reverse situation may occur when the worker is confronted by the saccharin-sweet, quiet patient, who denies discomfort or illness even when it is obvious that he is very uncomfortable or very ill. If the worker is the product of a volatile family life, he may see this patient as a "delight," one who doesn't seem to have a care in the world and whose concerns are minor. The worker may spend a great deal of time socializing at the bedside but, again, never thinks in terms of what is behind the facade presented by the patient.

The worker who has been reared by people he considers "normal" will probably use them as the basis for his perception of normality in others. The authoritarian father, the dependent mother, the selfless sister, the strong brother may be acceptable to the worker; while the dependent father, the authoritarian mother, the selfish sister, and the weak brother are not. He does not look at the patient's situation and evaluate it for itself, but rather is judgmental in terms of his own upbringing.

Health workers must be aware of their own physical and emotional state when approaching a patient. Anger at a coworker, worry about an ill family member, or such physical illness as a cold or an arthritis attack may result in a preoccupied, angry, or pained facial expression which the patient may think reflects the worker's response to his actions. It is wiser for the worker to postpone giving care—when this is feasible—or to explain to the patient that certain extenuating circumstances are causing his appearance of distress, rather than to allow the patient to feel that he is at fault.

Because cultures differ widely, they affect the worker's approach to a patient. One who enters an old-fashioned Japanese home without removing his shoes is regarded as uncouth. Yet walking shoeless into an American mansion would be equally unacceptable. Recognizing, accepting, and acting within cultural determinants help prevent the worker from developing misconceptions of patient behavior, and thus help establish a therapeutic atmosphere. The patient who senses that the worker lacks respect for his values is unlikely to establish a feeling of rapport with the worker. For example, a physician who conducted a filmed psychiatric family therapy session in a black patient's home, complained later that the family had not been amenable to therapy. He felt that they resented him because he was white, middle class, and Jewish. A review of the film supplied the real answer. The physician and his cotherapist had taken off their jackets and ties before being seated, and were blowing billows of cigar smoke through the well-kept living room. Meanwhile, the nonsmoking family stiffly maintained the formal appearance they normally exhibited in their most important room. The physician was unaware that his behavior, attire, and smoking were being regarded as signs of disrespect.

Religious beliefs that are different from those of the health worker are sometimes cited to explain one's inability to establish rapport with a patient, or as a reason for disliking or not understanding a patient. For example, staff members often show their anger at the "stupidity" of a severe cardiac patient who has refused to disavow religious scruples about birth control and who has become pregnant. The unkind remarks they make have their roots in religious bigotry. "Why not try self-control if you can't use birth control?" "Put a television set in your bedroom." "Don't you ever stop to think about the lack of natural supplies if the population continues to explode?" The patient may smile uncomfortably in her embarrassment, too upset to discuss her fear that she may not live long enough to raise her children and her even greater fear of perdition if she practices birth control.

The staff may also become furious with diabetic Jewish patients who insist on insulin that comes only from kosher animals. It becomes troublesome to exchange the medication on hand even when the other is easily accessible. The request ties in with the picture of "that demanding Jew," and does not take into account his training in regard to important religious observances.

The worker, too, may have to face expressions of intolerance. "I usually don't like blacks, but you're different." Such a remark by a patient may make the worker wonder, "Why should I help nurse this person back to health?" The worker has to accept the statement as one born of ignorance, and may safely counter it with, "Aren't all people different? Shouldn't each of us be judged for his personal worth rather than race, creed, or color?" If the worker speaks calmly, and without rancor, the patient may recognize his prejudices and start to review them. If the worker becomes angry, and storms out of the room, the patient will likely become indignant at the action of "that arrogant, lazy, stupid worker. I was only paying him a compliment."

Health workers find themselves changing in the face of constant involvement with patients who are suffering. Some are frightened at the thought of having a close emotional relationship with a patient, particularly one who may die, because the pain the worker will then go through may seem too much to bear. To avoid that pain, he remains detached, perhaps repeating incidents in the relationship that can be regarded humorously, but disregarding those which indicate the patient's suffering. To some, such a detached attitude is "professional." But is it? It is certainly not professional to avoid responding to the cry of the patient for a meaningful human relationship.

Assuming a facade of caring only for the specific "illness" of the patient may lead to feelings of guilt on the part of the worker. Although the patient may have a diseased gallbladder, his entire being is not encompassed by that organ. In fact, that aspect of his being may be minor in comparison to his view of himself in relation to others. The health worker who has empathy, and listens to the patient's complaints or problems, no matter how unrelated to his present illness, can provide a great deal of support. If he does more than just empathize and becomes involved (again we stress, not incapacitated), he can help the patient adjust to his life situation, or to make changes in his behavior that reflect new insights.

Some health workers have a compulsion to be the *total* supplier of all care to the patient. This attitude is often born of an inner need to be totally in control at all times. It does not take the needs or desires of the patient or family into consideration. This kind of worker does not allow the patient to plan any part of his care—his bathing, eating, sleeping, and recreational activities are all predetermined by the worker. For example: a mother "interferes" if she stays with her child; an adolescent is "disturbing to others" when quietly seated at a patient's bedside; anyone who receives special visiting privileges because he cannot come during the designated hours is met with hostility, and the visit will be interrupted for checking the patient's temperature or blood pressure, or for giving special treatments; the chronic patient is discharged without the needed practice in self-care, and is made to feel that he cannot possibly make decisions or do things for himself.

At the other end of the continuum is the worker who is anxious to relieve himself of responsibility for the patient. One nurse considered herself fortunate to be assigned to the care of a child with leukemia, because the mother remained in the room almost around the clock. The nurse would bring the bath supplies, linen, meals, and medications into the room, and say to the mother, "If you need anything, just call." She did not offer to care for the child, or speak to the mother or child about their feelings or problems. She was happy that she did not have to watch the child going downhill. She kept her distance, fearing any emotional involvement. She was unprepared for the mother's angry outburst when the child came nearer to death. "Of course I have to be here all the time! If I weren't, who would bathe, dress, or feed my child? No one takes any interest in us . . . no one cares." The nurse's own anxiety had been so high that she had failed to recognize the needs of the mother. It would have been far better if the mother had been relieved of responsibility for the child's nursing care, but had been allowed to work along *with* the nurse if she so desired. The mother would have then felt more confidence in the availability and competence of nursing care, and the child would have had a chance to develop rapport with the nurse. Then both mother and child might have been able to express their worries to the nurse, thereby easing their tensions.

A patient who bears great responsibility for others (a sick spouse, elderly parents, young children) is usually greatly admired by the hospital staff because his anxiety is ostensibly centered not on himself, but on the welfare of others, a trait that inspires admiration as well as sympathy. One patient was frantically worried about her blind diabetic husband, who in three sightless years had become totally dependent upon her. "Who will take care of him if I die?" "What will happen if I have to stay in the hospital for a long time?" The staff looked upon this woman as being full of virtue, always extending herself in consideration of her husband. Their own standards for being a "good" wife blinded them to a major fact—the patient had needlessly relegated her husband to the role of helpless invalid, even unable to pour a cup of coffee for himself. He, in turn, felt emasculated, but blamed his resulting sexual impotence on his diabetes. (Although this disorder is frequently associated with impotence, the patient's emotional reaction to his feelings of helplessness was the much larger factor.) The patient was helped to find practical solutions for her worries. A worker at a local institution for the blind went to the patient's home and taught the husband the necessary elements of self care. A college-aged son, still living at home, was happy to learn that he could help his father. Finally, the wife was able to speak to the hospital staff about her past hidden resentment at always having to be "the strong one." She also talked about her feelings of guilt when her husband developed the diabetic retinopathy that caused his blindness. "Maybe if I had been stricter about his diet, it wouldn't have happened." Had the staff not been so overwhelmed initially by the patient's "goodness," she might have received the help she needed sooner.

At times, the hospital worker may feel outranked by patients who are better educated than himself and avoid any meaningful discussion with such patients in order not to reveal his lack of education. The patient is then isolated, unable to have his needs met, simply because the needs of the worker to maintain his own prestige block any exchange. For example, a nurse may have been graduated from a diploma program, an associate degree program, or a baccalaureate program. Small wonder then that even an experienced nurse who has had little advanced education shudders at the thought of caring for the nursing director who holds a doctoral degree. Yet, if she can look at the patient as a human being who has all the hopes, worries, loves, and disappointments that other people have, rather than as the holder of a superior degree, she may be able to overcome her anxiety and provide empathic care that is also technically superior.

As the health worker gains experience, he has the opportunity to refine his techniques. If he wants to be more effective, he must evaluate what he is doing, and how it affects the patient. He will learn as much from his failures as from his successes, but only if he can truthfully assess his own contribution to both. He should evaluate the image he has projected—has he been directorial, permissive, judgmental, hostile, seductive, or concerned? How have the patients reacted? Would another approach have been more therapeutic? Was the worker meeting the needs of patients, or was he forcing them to meet the needs of the staff? Should the worker have called in a consultant more often?

If the worker has the interests of the patient at heart, he will be aware of the roles of other disciplines. Just as the physician asks the nurse to give the enema that he orders, so the nurse should feel free to call in the clinical nurse specialist, social worker, psychologist, physiotherapist, or home care expert. Each discipline has much to contribute to the patient's well-being, yet each has limitations. Working harmoniously as a team helps promote better care for the patient.

Since no one knows everything, it may be necessary to consult with others of one's own discipline to ensure the best possible patient care. The obstetric patient with heart disease may be assigned to a bed in the maternity division of the hospital, but she and her husband may benefit from a cardiac teaching program given in the medical division. Being aware of available programs and liaison personnel increases the scope of the worker's proficiency. If he limits himself to his own field, and remains unaware of the possibilities of utilizing help that can be given by personnel from other areas, he may also not become aware of the divergent needs of the patient. It is an unfortunate fact that when the worker does not recognize his own limitations he also is unable to see a need for outside consultation. Occasionally, workers who do know of other programs do not arrange for patient participation because they fear that the patient will think less of them for seeking outside assistance. In such a case, the worker needs help in defining priorities—which is more important: the needs of the patient or the worker's fear of a possible loss of status?

On occasion, the beliefs of the worker and those of the patient may clash, with tragic results. A patient who had experienced several severe postpartum depressions became pregnant although she had used a contraceptive. The patient, her husband, and the physician agreed that termination of the pregnancy was the only solution. The patient was assigned to a room on the maternity floor near the nursery, because the admitting officer could not "tie up a gynecology bed for this." A nurse told the patient, "I can't take care of you because abortion is against my religion." The anesthesiologist said, "I have to receive my fee in advance. You people leave the hospital very quickly." Although the patient was in therapy, she had to be rehospitalized for her severe depression and guilt following the procedure. Each staff member was either disinterested or unaware of how his statements would affect the patient.

In another case, a brilliant octogenarian who had been a practicing psychologist was losing her hearing, her sight, and her financial resources. She resented her dependence upon others, and withdrew any association with staff and other hospital residents whom she had difficulty in seeing and hearing. She looked forward to death, and frequently discussed her positive feelings about euthanasia for those who no longer wish to live. Staff members become very uncomfortable when she talked about euthanasia, a concept unacceptable to them. They described the patient as "haughty. . . . She thinks she's better than any of us." They overtly rejected her, and repeatedly placed her in the position of having to ask for help. One night, she encased herself in a sheet, and set herself on fire with her cigarette lighter. Staff members rushed in, beat out the flames, resuscitated her heroically, and spent long months treating her burns. When she was well enough, she was transferred to a state mental institution. After all, her suicidal attempt was a sign that she was crazy, wasn't it? Not one staff member had seen the need for intervention during the time that the patient was was talking about euthanasia and isolating herself from others. Instead, they looked upon her ideas and withdrawal as a hurtful, unacceptable rejection of themselves.

The health worker who can look upon himself honestly, taking credit for his virtues and trying to improve his shortcomings, will be able to care for his patients more effectively. The worker whose insecurity is too great to let him evaluate his own abilities and actions truthfully will be so anxious to protect himself that he will not hear patients' cries for help.

Fear of the patient's behavior may also hinder the thinking and actions of the worker. Occasionally, patients become assaultive, either because of a basic psychotic condition or a precipitating factor such as electrolyte imbalance. Several days after extensive intestinal surgery, a patient who had previously been quiet and who was later found to have such an imbalance, started screaming that the patient across the room was going to kill her. In defense, she threw everything she could get her hands on toward the other patient. Fortunately, her aim was very poor, and there were no injuries. The nurses who were on duty ran to the other patient to protect her, and themselves, from the onslaught. Only one nurse was unafraid. She walked directly to the patient and in a calm voice said, "No one will hurt you. I am beside you and will see to that." Hearing this, the patient reached out and grasped the nurse's hand. Within a short while she relaxed, and fell asleep. Had the nurse not been able to approach her, the assaultive behavior probably would have continued and even increased.

Workers also become fearful when patients harm themselves along with others. One psychotic patient would start her assaultive behavior in the day room. After shouting a long line of expletives, she would start throwing whatever was available, sending other patients, and often the staff, running for help. As they disappeared, she would look for smoldering cigarette butts dropped by patients, and burn her arms or legs with them. One day a nurse who had noted this pattern walked quickly to the patient when she started to curse aloud and calmly said, "I am not going to let you hurt yourself today." The patient screamed more foul language, and reached for a nearby ash tray. The nurse quickly maneuvered it away, saying, "I am not going to let you throw things, either." The nurse then extinguished the cigarette butt which the patient had thrown to the floor. At this, the patient screamed, "I hate you, I hate you, you no good _____." She banged her fists on the wall and began to sob. The nurse stood near by, not speaking or moving. Finally, the patient sat down on the couch, and the nurse sat near her. "I couldn't let you hurt yourself. I know how angry you feel, but there are other ways to get it out of your system." The patient did not seem to hear what was being said, but continued to sit on the couch, staring ahead. After a long silence she whispered, "You're a nice lady." After this episode, she continued to exhibit assaultive behavior on occasion, but never when that nurse was on duty.

This nurse, instead of showing fearfulness at the patient's actions, tried to understand what those actions meant. Thus she was able to empathize with the patient, and help in calming her down. Had the nurse become fearful, she might have tried to physically control the patient, an impossible task in view of the patient's greater strength and agility.

It may take time and experience for the worker to overcome his apprehension about working with difficult patients. However, if he expends his energies toward understanding why the patient is behaving in an unacceptable manner, rather than concentrating on his own fear, he is more likely to be effective in the situation.

The Use of the Interview

Should a staff member approach a patient who is known to have a problem? Some workers fear that their intervention will increase the patient's difficulty, and adversely affect the course of his illness. This rarely happens, for the patient can almost always accept anyone who is concerned, interested, and truthful. His emotional disturbance did not start with the worker's presence, but may be substantially decreased by it.

An interview is a conversation on a professional level. Peplau[1] notes that it has several purposes, including the *orientation* of the worker and the patient to each other, the *identification* of the patient's problems, and the *resolution* or institution of means to solve those problems. It differs from an ordinary conversation in that its function is not to provide socialization (except when that is a therapeutic goal) and it is usually planned for set times and places on a regularly scheduled appointment basis. The full time allotted for the appointment is kept by the worker whether or not the patient is present or responsive.

Orientation is the first step in establishing rapport with the patient. The worker greets the patient by name, and introduces himself by name and title. He then seats himself nearby, and tells the patient why he has come. "I understand that you are unhappy about your care," or "I have been called because you asked to speak to someone about your problems," or "How are things going?" The approach should be friendly but matter-of-fact, so that the patient does not feel as though he is going to be judged,

1. H. Peplau, *Interpersonal Relations in Nursing,* (New York: G. P. Putnam's Sons, 1952) pp. 17–42.

as he might if the interviewer appeared stern or threatening. If his anxiety level is high, he may not hear the introduction and will ask the interviewer to repeat his name, title, and the purpose of his visit. He may, in fact, request this information several times. "What did you say your name was again?" . . . "What do you do?" . . . "Why are you here?" If the worker realizes that anxiety and not inattentiveness is preventing the patient from hearing the answers, the situation will be more comfortable for all concerned. The worker should continue to repeat the answers in a friendly, matter-of-fact way, without showing any sign of annoyance.

Orientation may also focus upon the patient's stated desire for help. The fact that he recognizes his need for help is a step in the right direction, even though his perception of the actual problem may be distorted. The interview can then proceed to the next stage, that of identifying the problem.

Identification of the real problem is not always easy. The patient may focus on one symptom or event, and be unaware of what is really troubling him. It is up to the professional to listen carefully to what the patient is saying in order to discover the real problem. At times, the patient may shift the conversation to a different subject as the real difficulty starts to become apparent. He may become restless, say he is too tired to continue the interview, or develop a sudden pain that requires medication. These signs should alert the worker to the fact that the patient cannot tolerate further discussion along that line of inquiry. The patient may direct the conversation to safer subjects or remain silent, in which case the worker should just sit quietly until the end of the appointment. Before he leaves, the worker should tell the patient the time and place for the next interview, and that he will be available to the patient for as long as the patient remains in the hospital.

Resolution of the problem often follows its identification. Once the patient has been able to recognize what is really at the core of his trouble, he can usually think it through and reach a solution that is satisfactory to *him*. This is not to say that it would be acceptable to another patient in a comparable situation. Nor is it necessarily the ideal solution in the eyes of the worker. The important factor is that it meets the needs of the patient. If it is unsuccessful when tried, the patient should be helped to think the problem through again and to find alternate solutions, one of which may be more helpful.

A nurse consultant was called to see a patient who suddenly began to cry hysterically four days after having had a complete hysterectomy. She greeted the patient by name, introduced herself, sat down so that she could be on eye level with the patient, and said, "Would you like to talk about why you are crying so uncontrollably?" The patient nodded "yes" and continued to sob. In an attempt to help identify the problem, the nurse then said, "Sometimes women worry about the effects of this type of operation. They're afraid that it may affect their femininity." The patient shook her head from side to side, still crying and blowing her nose.

Between sobs, the patient finally said, "I'm a very sexy woman, and I've been looking forward to this so that I won't have to be concerned about becoming pregnant, or be annoyed by menstrual periods. It's not that. I just don't understand why I can't stop crying. It's been going on for six hours. I'm exhausted, but I can't get myself to stop." More tears, more nose blowing, more convulsive sobs.

The nurse sat silently for a while, then said quietly, "Many people anticipate dying during surgery, and cry afterwards for the sheer relief of being alive and on the way to recovery."

At this, the patient suddenly stopped crying, broke into a broad smile, and blurted, "That's it—I'm alive and I'm so relieved. I'm really alive!" By identifying her problem she had resolved it and her crying ceased.

A man who was scheduled for surgery to remove a cancer became depressed two days before surgery, refused to leave his bedside, and cried at intervals. Although his depression was understandable in light of the diagnosis, it seemed to be based on something more than that. The nurse consultant greeted him, introduced herself, and sat down near him. "The nurses tell me that you are very sad. Perhaps it would be helpful if you could share your feelings."

The patient's eyes filled with tears, and the nurse handed him a tissue. "I guess you must think I am not much of a man for crying." The nurse assured him that being a man was not at all dependent on whether or not one cried. "You know, I'm going to have a big operation, and the doctor says he can't tell how I'll be after it's over. I just don't know what to do."

The nurse said, "It's hard to face surgery when there are so many unfinished pieces of business to be completed." At this, the patient bowed his head and shoulders, and began to cry aloud.

"I've hurt so many people—everyone that I've loved. I lost my wife's money in the stock market, I stole from my best friend in business and, worst of all, I've antagonized my daughter so that she refuses to see or speak to me. I'm no good to anyone, not even to myself."

The patient went into each of these reasons for his depressed state in great detail. Losing his wife's money and stealing from his business partner were rash acts in a desperate bid for needed cash; his fight with his daughter involved her new husband. The patient believed that it was unmanly to apologize, and had therefore stopped communicating with his wife, his best friend, and his daughter. Now he needed to reopen those lines of communication in order to find inner peace. He finally decided that it was more important to ask each of them for forgiveness than to maintain his self-image of an unrelenting man. Although the reunions were tearful, they helped him resolve his inner conflicts. As soon as the stress of his emotional turmoil was relieved he was able to hold his head high again and face the surgery "like a man." His depression had lifted and he became hopeful about the outcome of the operation.

During any interaction, the worker must listen attentively to what the patient doesn't say, as well as to what he says. Sometimes unspoken words are more revealing than those which are said aloud. One young patient discussed his work history in great detail, but skipped over a five-year span during which he had worked for his father. Towards the end of that time, the situation at work had become so distressing that the son could neither sleep nor eat, and finally had to be admitted to a mental institution for three months. Another patient did not mention or recall his daughter's serious bout with rheumatic fever years before, but ruminated at length about the car he had purchased just before she became ill. A young woman who told a nurse that she was afraid to go home because she might harm her children and herself, was later unable to remember uttering that statement.

In some instances, communication is impeded because the patient speaks in a language of his own which is not understandable to anyone else. The interviewer should not permit such words and phrases to pass unchallenged since the patient may interpret this as a sign that he is being understood, or that the worker lacks real concern for him, or that he considers the patient "too crazy" to talk to. Pronouns may be misused (the patient may refer to himself as "he" rather than "I"), and neologisms (jargon coined by the patient) may hide the patient's thoughts. The worker can sometimes assess the meaning of confusing phrases by asking the patient to explain them as well as individual words that may be unclear. Unless both interviewer and patient have the same understanding of the patient's language, the patient's private world will remain impenetrable.

The patient who is totally mute is also communicating with the worker. His very silence becomes a challenge, since the worker must then try to unravel the mystery of this nonverbal communication. It may be difficult to tolerate the silence, to realize that it is part of the patient's illness. Spending time with the patient reassures him that he is a worthy person. Although silent, he realizes that he is communicating with you if you meet his physical needs by intuitively providing care that his body gestures suggest (offering him food if he seems hungry, a drink if his lips appear parched). In time, he may feel free enough to start communicating on a verbal level. However, coaxing him to do so before he is ready will increase his need to remain mute.

Listening to what a patient says during an interview involves more than just hearing the spoken words. The *content* of the discussion may only tangentially refer to the subject matter that the patient really wants to talk about. He may be fearful of his ability to deal with the matter once it is exposed, of being ridiculed, or of losing his status in the worker's eyes if the material is ludicrous or unsavory.

The worker must also be aware of the patient's mood during the interview. The patient may exhibit sadness, tearfulness, happiness, or anxiety which may be appropriate to the content of the interview. At other times, the affect (mood) may be totally out of context. The patient who smilingly tells the worker about a long series of disastrous happenings is reacting inappropriately.

As the interviewer listens to the content, his mind may rush ahead, trying to decide what is important, and what material has hidden meanings. The patient may begin to discuss his fight to get a hot cup of coffee with breakfast. The worker may sympathetically jump in to agree with the fact that coffee just never seems to arrive hot at the bedside. Actually, the patient's main concern was the fight, not the coffee. Each employee she asked had promised to bring in a fresh, hot cup of coffee, and each disappeared without doing so. If no one could meet that simple request, how could they be trusted to care for her following complicated abdominal surgery?

Sometimes a worker will sidetrack the patient when an item of common interest is brought up. The patient may start to discuss something that happened on a camping trip. The interviewer, also a camper, may say, "Oh, you enjoy camping, too. Where have you gone? What type of camper did you use?" The events that the patient wanted to bring up are lost in meaningless socialization.

Frequently, patients will direct personal questions at the interviewer, asking whether he is married, has children, lives nearby, and so on. If the worker feels comfortable in doing so, he may answer the questions briefly, without going into detail, and quickly switch the focus back to the patient. "I appreciate your interest in whether I am married. Perhaps your basic concern is whether a single person could help you with some marital problem?" This brings up the fact that the worker understands that the patient is uneasy and has mixed feelings about talking and revealing himself. It also acknowledges the patient's curiosity about the worker's competence and knowledgeableness.

If the patient says, "Somehow, you remind me of my mother," the worker can use that by saying, "In what way?" or "Describe her to me." The patient can then proceed to discuss whatever he wishes, since either phrase can refer to physical, emotional, vocational, educational, or other aspects of the patient's mother that are brought to mind.

The interviewer may find notes on the patient's chart that describe some behavior problem. Relatives or friends may also want to talk to the worker to share bits of information. Some workers like to read the chart and speak to others first, so as to have as much prior knowledge about the patient as is available. Other interviewers prefer to speak to the patient first, and not be "contaminated" by the reports and remarks of others. If the latter course is taken, the worker may seek other information later in order to get a picture of the patient and to clarify what the patient has said.

A patient who was terminally ill with cancer and who suddenly became very depressed furnishes a case in point. Ostensibly, she was concerned about the fact that she would not be able to meet the expenses incurred by her illness. In a series of interviews, she brought up the changes that had occurred in her life since her husband's death several years earlier. She spoke of him in endearing terms, and told of how admired he was by everyone who knew him. Suddenly, her face reddened in anger. "Everyone, that is, but me! He never planned ahead for me. He spent everything he earned and didn't have much insurance. He changed jobs just two years before he died, and lost the pension and other benefits that he had accumulated. After he died, I had to go to work. I wasn't trained for anything, and had to lie about my age and qualifications to get a job. It all worked out, but I hate him for putting me in such a position." She went on to tell of her difficulties in getting along with her daughter, and of her son's marital difficulties and divorce.

The notes on the chart indicated that the patient was always cooperative and pleasant, and that she stressed her desire to "not be a burden" to anyone. Although too weak to be out of bed without help, she went to the bathroom alone one night, fell, and injured herself. She was very apologetic to all the staff members involved in getting her back to bed. The next day, a deep depression set in.

The daughter described her mother as "authoritarian." "She just won't let go. I'm almost 40 years old, and she still tells me how to dress, and how to live, and how to raise my two children. She's loved by everyone who knows her, but [and here she began to cry] I hate her. She has always made my brother the good one, and me the bad one. I won't have her in my home because she causes trouble between my husband and me. I can't help being angry with her, or feeling guilty about it later."

With all this information, the interviewer was able to help the patient look at her illness and its effects from a different angle. The worry about finances was only a ploy to disguise her anguish about losing control over herself and her daughter. Slowly, she was able to bring out her fear of becoming dependent upon others. The interviewer discussed this problem with the staff who responded by giving the patient as much latitude in determining her own care as possible. Medications for pain were adjusted in consultation with her. She wanted relief, but did not want to be drowsy so much of the time. Smaller doses were given more frequently, until a happy medium was met. The patient was also urged to dictate her dietary preferences, and to decide upon times for her personal care. All of these steps contributed towards lessening her sense of dependency.

In further interviews, the worker discovered that the patient had always resented the close relationship between her husband and their daughter, and had remained aloof from her daughter because she sensed she would be rejected. Instead she developed close ties with her grandchildren, who loved her dearly. Gradually, as she explored her feelings, she lessened her attempts at control over her daughter, thus easing the strain between the two of them. Before she died, they were able to spend pleasant hours together, learning about each other, and gaining some of the closeness that each wanted through the years.

To be effective, the interviewer must remain nonjudgmental, regardless of what he is told. This was particularly true in the mother-daughter interviews cited above. Had the worker sided with either the mother or the daughter (or the son or dead husband) he could not have helped in the resolution of the patient's problems. By maintaining himself outside the realm of the problem, he was able to help both the patient and her daughter work towards a solution.

Once a counseling relationship has started, an inexperienced worker and the patient may find that they have developed a close personal relationship. This becomes a problem if the patient wants to continue meeting the worker socially after he leaves the hospital. One way to prevent this is to make it clear during the orientation phase that the worker will be available *until* the patient is discharged from the hospital. As that time draws near, the worker should remind the patient of this. "I will be seeing you while you are still here in the hospital. After you leave, arrangements can be made for you to see someone else on an outpatient basis." This must be mentioned frequently, so that the patient will not interpret a rejection of social invitations as a rejection of himself. For the relationship to be therapeutic, the worker should not become involved socially with the patient at any time.

Respecting Confidentiality

Patients reveal a great deal about themselves during the time they are involved in interviews. Feelings that they perhaps have not admitted even to themselves may suddenly come to the surface. They must be assured with certainty that anything they share with the interviewer will be held in confidence. This is imperative, since confidentiality is a prime concern, particularly when the discussion involves actions, thoughts, or feelings that might be embarrassing to the patient.

Information that the patient discloses must be regarded as privileged and must not be bantered about by hospital or agency personnel not directly involved in the patient's care. If the team approach is being used, every member of the team is obligated to respect totally and absolutely the information that is revealed by the worker in conferences. As a professional person, the worker's ethics should prevent him from divulging information about patients to neighbors, friends, or family, even though the patient is not known to them. In fact, discussion of confidential material is unethical even though the worker is away from the clinical setting, and feels certain that the patient is not identifiable.

Sometimes patients are so fearful of a breach of confidentiality that they will withhold pertinent information. In one instance, a Caucasian patient did not tell her physician that she had been having extramarital sexual relations with a supposedly sterile Chinese man. When her unknowing husband who believed he had impregnated his wife saw the oriental appearance of the newborn, he accused the hospital of switching babies. The wife was unwilling to divulge the truth about the baby's parentage until her husband initiated a lawsuit against the hospital. At that point, she told her husband the truth, asking him to drop the suit before the local newspapers printed the story. The marriage subsequently was terminated, with husband and wife each going into therapy.

What if the patient tells the interviewer that he is planning to commit suicide, or a homicide? Can confidentiality be respected in such an instance? What will happen to the relationship if the interviewer shares such information with others?

The worker should never agree to meet demands of the patient before he knows what prompts them. If the patient says, "I'll tell you what I'm planning if you promise that you won't tell anyone," the worker should reply sincerely, "I can't help you fully unless I know what is really bothering you. I never make promises I can't keep. It wouldn't be fair to either of us. Furthermore, such a promise might make me incapable of giving you the kind of care and attention most beneficial to you."

When a patient discusses committing an act of violence, he is crying for help. He is afraid that he will not be able to control his impulses without outside assistance. The worker must then help him reach the point where he can discuss his intentions with his physician. The worker can support the patient and remain with him, but cannot accept the total responsibility for preventing an irresponsible action. He can say to the patient, "The fact that you are able to share this information indicates that you realize you need help. I am not in a position to offer all the assistance you need. Your doctor will be able to offer a wider range of suggestions than I. Until you speak with him, I shall try to help you in every way I can. It would be best if *you* speak to the doctor, rather than have me transmit your thoughts to him. How do you feel about this?"

Some workers find it difficult to respond in a professional manner if the patient rejects the suggestion that he confide in the doctor. If the worker himself has never been able to trust others, he may very well be adamant in his feeling that he should not disclose the patient's plans to anyone else. He reasons, "I wouldn't want anyone to interfere with my plans after I confided in him." His judgment is obviously impaired because of his feeling that what he would want for himself is best for the patient.

When the patient refuses to speak with the doctor, the interviewer should try to determine the reason. If the patient refuses to change his mind, the worker should state calmly and factually, "I guess I will have to speak to him, although it would be more meaningful if you did. It is important to me that you not be permitted to hurt yourself or others. The doctor can help in that effort."

The suicidal patient is often isolated and placed on certain precautions which may include locking the windows permanently, searching his belongings for dangerous implements, and keeping nurses at his bedside around the clock. One patient, in a riverside hospital, mulled over his rejections of various methods of committing suicide. "I'd jump out of the window, but I'm afraid of heights." "I'd jump into the river, but I can't swim." "I'd slash my wrists, but I can't stand the sight of blood." "I'd hang myself, but I can't stand anything tight around my neck." And so on, ad infinitum. It is important that staff members assigned to the patient share such information so that everyone can help protect the patient from himself.

Patients who are transferred from a psychiatric service to another area in a general hospital often worry about the reports that go with them. They should be assured that confidential information will not be placed on the chart, but that a note advising the staff of appropriate ways to care for them will be included.

Facts pertinent to the care and understanding of the patient may be shared with other staff members only if they understand and respect confidentiality. A patient's personal problems and motivations are not to be bandied about for the titillation of coworkers or friends. Health workers are legally responsible for confidentiality, and are liable for any unprofessional breach of that trust.

When a patient confides in the worker, the information must never be used to the worker's self-advantage. One worker became so interested in a patient's tales of her sexual prowess that he decided to test her skill for himself. The patient reported the seduction, noting that it was just one more affirmation of her belief that men were interested in her only for her body. Another worker became excessively attentive to a patient who told of his vast financial holdings. Her attention to this patient was noticed by the staff, and remarked upon by the patient who said, "She is probably after my money." Discussions with the worker revealed her plan to utilize the patient's acumen as a guide in her own financial dealings.

The staff must not use the patient's psychiatric status to intimidate him in any way. One health worker on a psychiatric unit told a patient that it didn't matter what the worker said to him, because "no one would believe a report from a nut." Fortunately, the patient did not allow himself to be intimidated, and reported the incident, which was then thoroughly investigated by the staff. Similar incidents were revealed by several other patients who had been afraid to say anything because they feared reprisals by the worker.

Often the change-of-shift report is a time when the staff gossip about the patient. This seems to relieve them of tensions accumulated during the tour of duty, but it is demeaning to the patient and prevents the formulation of more meaningful goals for his care. Noisy laughter and often total immersion of staff in stories about patients are sometimes overheard or observed by patients, who may then believe that their confidences are not kept. Although health workers are also human, they should not use staff conferences to denigrate patients who are, at the moment, less fortunate.

Telephones that workers use to discuss privileged information with the doctor or other professionals should be in a private area to prevent the conversation from being overheard. Often times the health worker uses a telephone that is centrally located, with the result that any patient who is nearby hears what is being said. This may cause the patient who overhears to lose confidence in the staff's ability to maintain confidentiality. Once that happens, the patient is unlikely to confide in any staff member again.

The Health Worker in the Community

When the health worker is knowledgeable about the extent of mental illness in this country, he realizes also that an awareness of the factors in prevention must become part of every health worker's armamentarium. The institution of treatment after mental illness has taken hold is not enough. It is imperative for all health workers to recognize those situations that may give rise to causative factors, so that the number of hospital beds allotted to psychiatric patients in the United States can be lowered from its present 50 percent level.

Prevention of mental illness can take place on three levels.[1] On the *primary* level, the health worker tries to prevent or alleviate situations that may contribute to mental health problems. Perhaps this can be accomplished by efforts to change the home, community, or work environment, or by helping people to anticipate and handle crises that are of maturational or situational origin. On the *secondary* level, the health worker strives for recognition, diagnosis, and early treatment of problems. On the *tertiary* level, the worker tries to prevent a worsening of the illness, while working towards rehabilitation of the patient. At times, workers find themselves involved with a patient on all three levels at one time. For example, the patient's illness may have been recognized and treatment instituted. During the same period, his work situation may require intervention. Meanwhile, rehabilitation is started with vocational training geared towards placing the patient in a less tension-creating job.

1. G. Caplan. *Principles of Preventive Psychiatry.* (New York: Basic Books, Inc., 1964).

Hospitalization for any mental illness should be for as short a time as possible. The patient should remain in the community whenever feasible, to prevent the additional problems that prolonged hospitalization often brings. Such problems often result from one's separation from home, friends, and work, and the development of a sense of hopelessness and a feeling of helplessness that comes from dependence on others for the gratification of every need and desire.

In a sense, everyone who has contact with another human being is a health worker. Neighbors, relatives, teachers, friends, shopkeepers, as well as social workers, nurses, psychologists, and physicians can recognize the beginnings of unhealthy behavior. Beauticians and bartenders are often privy to people's fears and anxieties long before any health professional is involved. It is the duty of the health worker to see that the public is made aware of community resources in the hope that they will be contacted if the need arises.

The public health nurse is in a unique position to uncover behavior patterns that indicate incipient psychiatric illness. Her excursions into homes permit her to see family exchanges that may be unhealthy. She may note that a certain member is the scapegoat for all family problems, or that another is the troublemaker, or that still another lashes out inappropriately in anger. She may hear unrealistic expectations, and note flights into unreality to escape those expectations. She may relate poor school performance to an intolerable home situation. If she enters the home with the idea of giving care for one specific condition, and does not note situations that may be contributing to mental health problems in the patient or other family members, she is not performing her function to the fullest extent possible.

The public health nurse may also be active in schools or other institutions. She may be present to conduct eye tests, but notice signs of other problems in the children being tested. A child may have a severe tic, lack control of bladder and bowel function, fall asleep in class, or show signs of drug abuse. If the nurse focuses all her energies on the eye tests, she will not be aware of these other signs of incipient psychiatric problems.

Social workers also have the opportunity to note problems as they are presented in patients' homes or in institutions. Although a worker may ostensibly be present to assess the need for public assistance, he may find a family in acute distress because of the illness of the breadwinner. The father may have become totally dependent, both physically and emotionally, on the mother. He may terrorize the children, or remain silent and withdrawn. The children may not understand what is happening, and attribute his illness and its effects to their own "badness" or "bad" thoughts. If the mother then tells them, "Be quiet, or you'll make daddy worse," they may be overwhelmed by the thought that their father's recovery rests on their ability to be quiet. Again, financial assistance may seem to be *the* problem to the social agency, while actually it is minor in terms of family mental health.

A child's schoolteacher may be the first to recognize his physical or emotional problems. He notes that a child who has never spent much time in the bathroom suddenly starts to urinate frequently, and is drinking copious amounts of fluid. The teacher may assume that the child is trying to avoid classwork, while the youngster may really be showing the first signs of diabetes. Another child may seem to doze off for a few seconds at a time, or be unaware of what is happening around him. He may be having petit mal episodes. Still another may find it difficult to concentrate on his studies, and may not be working up to his potential. The teacher may automatically label him as "lazy," or, on the other hand, he may investigate and find that certain definite factors are causing the child's behavior. Teachers can be excellent case finders, as the two following case reports indicate.

Eight-year-old Joey's teacher urged the child's mother to ask for help from a neighborhood mental health center because the boy had begun to wet himself frequently in class. The mother told the nurse at the center that the child had also recently become enuretic, and that she was disgusted with him. He was the second of five children, and had been born seven months after her husband committed suicide rather than wait for inevitable death from acute leukemia. She had not been able to care for Joey during his infancy, and had placed both Joey and his older brother in a series of foster homes for two years.

The mother regarded her husband's suicide as an insult to herself. If he had really loved her, he would have waited to see the outcome of her pregnancy. To help regain her sense of being desirable, she had entered into a series of romantic alliances that had resulted in three more children. The father of the youngest child wanted to marry her, but she felt his unstable work record was a drawback. He lived in the home sporadically, but would leave when he was out of work and unable to contribute financially.

Joey appeared very bright, and tested well on standard IQ tests. The mother wanted him to be the "best" student in his class, and envisioned him as going to college in the future. She placed great pressure on him to do his schoolwork, and forbade friendships with neighborhood youngsters, whom she considered beneath him both intellectually and socially. His only companion was the next younger brother, a year his junior.

Although the mother qualified for public assistance, she refused it as degrading. She held a full-time job, and delegated household tasks to be completed by the three older children before she came home from work. (The two youngest were cared for by a neighbor.) None were allowed to leave the house or backyard after returning from school, or to invite playmates to the house because the mother looked upon other children as a possible contaminating source of bad habits, such as drug abuse or other antisocial behavior.

In describing his life, Joey said he didn't know how to make friends, and that he spent all his time studying. He looked sad as he described doing poorly in some subjects because he was afraid to ask the teacher for explanations. He wanted to join a Boy Scout troop, but his mother would not permit it when she was told she would have to be available for some activities. "It probably wouldn't have been any good anyway!" As for wetting, "I just get that feeling and then it happens . . . like I'm scared, and I don't know what to do . . . when the teacher calls on me, and I don't know the answer . . . when my mother yells at us, and says she hates us and she's leaving us forever."

Meetings with the mother revealed her erratic temper. She found that she could get the children to behave if she stormed out of the home in a rage, and did not come back for several hours. "I'm afraid I'll kill them when I get very angry." She had been unaware of their terror that she really would never come back. "I thought they knew I was kidding." As she talked with the nurse, she decided to try a new pattern of behavior. Instead of raging when angry, she would force herself to talk to the children about what made her angry, but would no longer threaten to leave home. The children learned to change their behavior when she would say, "I am getting furious." Joey in particular began to relax when the threat of desertion lessened.

The visiting nurse went to the school and spoke to the young, dynamic teacher who had made Joey her special project. The teacher was anxious to have him succeed, and recognized that he was hampered by insecurities. "I made him the monitor in charge of homework so that he would realize how much I think of him. He has to check everyone's notebook and report those who have not done their work." She was aware of his inability to make or maintain friendships, and asked the nurse for help in this area. The nurse helped her to understand Joey's role as homework monitor as seen by the other youngsters. Since many of them did not do their assignments, he was regarded as responsible for getting them into trouble. He was torn between his desire to stay on their good side and his responsibility to the teacher. She was concerned by the stress she had unwittingly caused with her well-intentioned appointment. She decided to talk with Joey, and offer him a choice of two other tasks instead—he could either become the monitor who distributed milk, or the one who controlled the window shades. He chose the latter since "some kids don't like milk, but everyone likes the sun out of his eyes."

The teacher also devised some games in which the children worked sequentially with different classmates in twosomes. Joey was thus able to widen his one-to-one contacts in the class. He befriended a new pupil who spoke only Spanish, and took great pride in being able to teach him some English. Although he did not form any close friendships with any of the other children, he began to feel more comfortable with them.

The mother discussed her expectations for Joey with the teacher and admitted to the pressure he was under to do both his schoolwork and household tasks. The teacher then realized that her own tactics in forcing him to produce were adding to the overwhelming pressure from home and decided to lessen her demands on him. "Even if he is bright enough to go on to college, they won't take him if he's still wetting himself!"

Joey's physical appearance changed as he felt less pressure. His shoulders were less stooped, and he smiled occasionally. His voice, which had been almost inaudible, became louder and firmer. He stopped wetting himself, both day and night. Although his mother still would not allow him any social contacts after school, he found it easier to be friendly with others at lunchtime and during recess periods.

The nurse at the mental health center met with Joey weekly during this time. At first, he sat on a chair several feet away, and kept his eyes averted. He would take a very large doll from the shelf, and talk to it. "You know you have to keep clean. . . . I'm not going to wash your wet things. . . . What do you mean you were in trouble in school?" As time went on, he no longer needed the doll, and could speak directly about his troubles. On occasion, he would cuddle up to the nurse. From the beginning of their relationship Joey was told that the nurse "will only be able to see you for three months."

When he was reminded that the time for termination of his interviews was near, Joey silently walked to the window, shoulders drooping, hands in his pockets and, with his back to the nurse, quietly said, "I guess that's what always happens when you find a friend. They leave you."

"But Joey, the things we learned from each other will always remind us of each other. Even though we won't be together each week, we have had the chance to really know each other, and that was good."

"I guess so."

"Remember when we first met? I told you we would only be together for three months. There's nothing either of us can do about the short time."

Joey wet himself in school and during the night several times the next week. Both his mother and teacher had been warned of this possibility, and did not fuss about it. Joey asked that the last visit between himself and the nurse take place in school. There, he gave the nurse an ornament which he had made for her. He asked her to walk into the hall with him, and said, "Could you give me a kiss goodbye, and then leave, fast, when I go back to the room? I don't want to say anything else." And so they parted. Joey's later history showed that he remained dry for the most part, and was more competent in school. Although he was more comfortable with others, he still avoided close friendships. It was hoped that as his mother would give him more freedom, this would change and he would find friendships that would last.

Ten-year-old Vivian had accused the school custodian of raping her. Physical examination determined that she had not been molested. The school principal was aware of the girl's seductive manner toward boys in her class, and suggested to the child's mother that she contact the neighborhood mental health center. After speaking with the mother, the nurse at the center determined that family therapy within the home would be most practical, since there were one older and three younger children to be cared for at home, making clinic visits on a regular basis unlikely.

The entire family looked forward to each session. The five children, mother, and her boyfriend usually sat in a circle in the same order: two-year-old, mother, twelve-year-old, four-year-old, seven-year-old, mother's boyfriend, patient, and the nurse. It soon became apparent that the patient was cut off every time she tried to speak. She was also blamed for all unpleasant family incidents. She initiated much dissension between the others, and was sexually provocative towards her mother's boyfriend.

Vivian's father had deserted his family after the last child was born. He was overwhelmed by his financial responsibility for five children. Although the boyfriend wanted to marry the mother, she refused, reasoning that by remaining unmarried she could continue to collect public assistance money.

As the oldest girl, Vivian was expected to help make beds, cook meals, and wash dishes, although not the pots. (The only other girl was the two-year-old.) She resented this, along with the fact that she was not given "grown up" freedom consistent with her household responsibilities.

Although she was often placed in charge of the younger children while her mother visited friends, she was punished if she chastised them. She was ambivalent about being the mother-substitute. She enjoyed the sense of being trusted, but disliked the limitations placed on her. The others said she was "too bossy" while in charge. They would often think up ways to get her into trouble. The mother always said that she "knew" Vivian was the troublemaker, even without investigating. She hated doing housework and reasoned that it was "good experience" for Vivian to take over certain tasks, pointing out that she herself did the two most hated tasks—washing the pots and cleaning the bathroom.

The mother placed restrictions on all her children's friendships. If she knew and approved of the outsiders, they could be invited to visit. However, only the oldest boy was permitted to visit other friends. Vivian resented not being given the same amount of freedom.

As arguments took place during the family therapy sessions, the behavior of various members became apparent, and this was discussed. The other youngsters began to realize how they were goading Vivian until she would lose control and become dictatorial. The mother decided to stop relying on Vivian for the major portion of the household tasks. Vivian in turn reacted to the easing of the pressures by calming down and not ordering others about. The school principal noted less seductive behavior in school, and an improvement in her work.

At the last family session, Vivian insisted that her mother sit near the boyfriend. Vivian was permitted her full say when she talked and remained in good control of herself. Her mother agreed to let her visit two girl friends after school and praised her for her help that day.

In each of the cases cited, initiation of treatment was suggested by members of school staffs. It is unlikely that either patient would have received help without the referral. Early recognition of the problems allowed the needed intervention before unacceptable behavior patterns became too deeply ingrained.

Unfortunately, neither school had a school nurse attached to it. School nurses should be assigned to develop health programs that will benefit both the school population and their families. Even though a teacher may notice abnormal behavior, he may be unable to get help for the child if the parent refuses to accept his recommendation. A school nurse could make a home visit and, because of her medical background, would be likely to recognize any unusual family patterns or problems which are contributing to the child's difficulty. Parents are more likely to accept her suggestion for seeking help, since she appears as an authority figure in the health field.

In many schools, the nurse is also responsible for individual health teaching and guidance. Information available to her about each child enables her to tailor programs to the needs of each. In a sense, she is the coordinator of health care for each child, collecting information from home, doctor, teacher, and community agencies that have contributed to the child's care. She sorts the information and shares appropriate sections with those who are involved with the child. She also makes referrals to mental health agencies if such care is required.

Community centers are another source of mental health referrals. Workers in charge of preschoolers can spot problems that may be due to retardation, lack of maturation, or environmental factors. Parents who are unaware of normal behavior patterns may either forgive or damn their children wrongfully. The normal "No" of the two-year-old may be very threatening to the authoritarian parent, while the abnormal clinging of her four-year-old may fill the need of an insecure mother. If the center holds group meetings for parents, these can be utilized for giving parents information about normal child development so they can become better prepared to deal with their children at all age levels.

In community centers that are available to school-age youngsters agency workers have an opportunity to note those who are overly aggressive and those who are loners, those who may be victims of child abuse, and those who are not reacting in acceptable fashion. The perceptive worker can then refer these children to suitable helping agencies. Teenagers often present problems, particularly in the areas of acting-out with drugs or sex, that come under the scrutiny of the center's workers. "Rap" sessions often help these young people to look at their life styles critically and, for some, this may be sufficient to cause them to cease the pursuit of unacceptable or harmful behavior. Others may need more personalized professional help to solve their problems. Identity crises are common at this age, and it is invaluable for community centers to have workers present who are trained to recognize such problems.

Golden Age clubs are another area in which community workers can be helpful in identifying the mental health needs of older people. Elderly people may exhibit signs of senile arteriosclerosis, and the forgetfulness and suspicion that accompany it may give rise to unsatisfactory home situations. Unless some social outlet is provided, older people tend to isolate themselves, and will not care for themselves properly. They may forget to eat, bathe, or take prescribed medications on time. Conversely, they may overeat, or take too much medication. The mental stimulation of being engaged in activities with others seems to slow the aging process. Gerontologists have noted that the elderly who work or are consistently mentally active are less likely to deteriorate.

Crises in living occur when an older person loses his mate, when his friends die, and when he may be forced to move in with one of his children. He resents the loss of his independence and of the familiarity of his own home. He may be unhappy at having to revise his schedule to fit that of a young family and may, in turn, sense the discomfort of children and grandchildren who loved him during short visits, but now find it hard to adjust to his permanent presence. Group sessions for these senior citizens may help ease their tensions. Sometimes members can arrange for joint living accommodations, thus providing themselves with compatible companions. Their families may also benefit from individual or group counseling available at the center or an associated agency.

The concerned health worker is also interested in milieu ecology. His efforts to improve community health extend beyond the individual to an involvement in society and active participation in change. He recognizes community problems that may contribute to illness, and works toward change. When illness is present among individuals in the community, the worker facilitates its treatment before it becomes ingrained, and plans for long-range care and rehabilitation. To do this, he must be familiar with local agencies and their referral systems. He should also be aware of any gaps in the provision of health services, and be actively seeking institution of missing services. He should be able to speak to community groups, in coordination with existing agencies, to make the community aware of its needs. He should be a resource person, able to help the community set priorities in meeting those needs and to suggest ways that funds can be used most beneficially for the community at large.

In an effort to utilize mental health facilities to the utmost, some communities have implemented day hospitals and night hospitals along with the usual custodial residences and outpatient clinics. These provide necessary services for patients who do not require full-time hospitalization, yet are unready or unable to live at home. Some patients can work during the day, yet need the security of the hospital situation at night. Others are able to spend the night at home, but need the structured situation of the hospital during the day. Providing both types of facilities releases inservice beds without denying appropriate services for the patient who is preparing to return to the community. A full range of therapeutic programs is available in both day and night hospitals, including individual and group sessions, vocational, recreational, and rehabilitation activities. Patients continue to use these services until they are able to manage on their own. Frequently, they are given an emergency telephone number which they may call at any time in the event they need immediate help.

Some communities have set up a crisis intervention center, with telephones manned twenty-four hours a day by individuals trained in crisis techniques. Patients who call are usually given appointments to be seen within twenty-four hours at a nearby clinic. (If the situation is acute, the patient may be seen immediately.) After the initial consultation, the patient is given a follow-up appointment or is hospitalized if necessary. Many colleges have set up such centers on their campuses. They are frequently manned by nurses, psychologists, or social workers who are in graduate school. The calls they receive are often tied in with drug abuse, unwanted pregnancy, or poor interpersonal relationships. When threats of suicide are received, immediate preventive action is instituted. Appointments are made as necessary for follow-up care in the hospital or community.

Health workers who are assigned to the community find that their responsibilities go far beyond their job descriptions. Those involved with families in ghetto slums may find themselves battling with landlords and governmental agencies to secure housing that meets even minimal standards, sufficient food, proper clothing, and necessary health care for their patients. At first, much of their time may be spent in determining what the community *wants* as well as what it needs. The worker may have determined the needs accurately, but if those needs do not coincide with what the community wants, the worker's efforts will be met with resistance. The astute worker will recognize the demand for autonomy by the people. A community's intense desire to determine its own fate without outside direction must be respected if the worker is to gain the trust of its residents.

The community health worker soon finds that it is important for him to become a member of local committees. In so doing, he emphasizes his desire to be part of the community and to play a role in its betterment. It is equally important, however, that he approach his committee work as a part of the team, that he listen to others and not try to take over the leadership. He will need to determine where the real power of the community lies and what lines of communication he can use to reach that person. Sometimes seemingly powerful leaders are merely fronts for the quiet sideliners who wield the true power. Convincing the sideliners may be the most effective way of gaining the "leader's" support for needed programs to be backed by the community. It may also be necessary for the worker to inform the leaders that there are programs, agencies, and other resources available to the community if they desire to take advantage of them. Such information implies that the worker is sharing his knowledge, not trying to make decisions for the community.

Preventive psychiatry depends upon the worker's competence in recognizing the interplay between the individual and his milieu. Workers must assess all aspects of the effects of environment on the individual, determine how these forces affect him, how he reacts to them, and what strengths he in turn brings into play against the environment. Unless the evaluation is complete and critical, important factors may be disregarded, and time wasted on trivia. To illustrate: Several years ago a severe earthquake in the Los Angeles area resulted in widespread evidence of emotional damage. Adults as well as children sought guidance in calming their fears. Many complained of feeling weak and helpless and of an inability to sleep after the disaster which had occurred in the middle of the night. Children wakened with fantasies about their parents fighting, apparently the result of feeling they had been shaken and punished. Many blamed such feelings on "bad thoughts." Mental health workers in the area encouraged the victims to discuss their experiences rather than allow their anxieties to remain pent up. Intervention took the physical effects of the disaster into account, including displacement from homes, schools, and work areas. It is unlikely that any other approach would have been effective in that situation.

Crisis Intervention

Health workers are often caught up in a patient's problems which may or may not be directly related to the condition for which he is being treated. The patient may vent his feelings in terms of the condition, while in reality his anxieties are based on problems that are not associated with it. For example, a teen-ager may lament her imperfect profile, and blame it for her lack of boyfriends, when her argumentative imperious manner is the real factor that drives boys away. The health worker can help such a patient explore the personality factors which are playing a part in alienating others. A determination of the real factors involved will, it is to be hoped, lead to the formulation of helpful solutions.

A *crisis* is a situation in which the usual balance in living is disturbed, and for which techniques used previously to solve problems are inadequate. Often a patient is suddenly beset by what seems to be an insurmountable problem. Under ordinary circumstances he may be able to cope well, but the additional pressure of a crisis situation immobilizes him. He must find new problem-solving techniques in order to find a solution to the problem and return to a state of equilibrium. Successful solutions may be based on past life experiences which turned out well; those which are unsuccessful may involve memories of unresolved problems that are in some way symbolized by the present conflict. The individual may continue in a state of disequilibrium until he can devise a solution that will allow him to cope adequately with the present situation. Intervention by trained professionals may be needed for this.

Crises occur throughout life as part of the growth process. Maturational crises may be dealt with in a variety of ways, depending upon the individual's ability to formulate and understand the problems, and his coping mechanisms. If he views a problem as insoluble because he cannot handle it by using his established problem-solving techniques, he will feel overwhelmed. He may become tense, anxious, or depressed as he fails to find a solution. In desperation, he may develop somatic complaints, regress in his behavior, or even withdraw from the situation into an unreal world in an effort to get away from the problem. Hopefully, correctly formulating the problem and deciding upon a solution will restore the individual to a state of equilibrium that is *higher* than his initial level of functioning. However, there are times when that level may only *equal,* or even be *lower,* than the level prior to the crisis.

Crises tend to last from one to six weeks. They may end by being resolved, redefined, or avoided through a change in the original goals. If none of these techniques has been successful, disequilibrium continues. When this happens, tensions rise, anxiety continues, and the patient may exhibit physical or behavioral symptoms which interfere with functioning.

Maturational crises start with birth. The birth process may be more hazardous for some than others, depending upon the intrauterine environment, genetic factors, and the relative proportions of the maternal pelvis and the neonate. The infant who reaches gestational maturity, has no defects, and goes through the birth process easily is better able to adapt to the external world. The child who is born prematurely, or has a birth defect, certainly faces a crisis as soon as he is born. He may have to be separated from the mother immediately and sent to an intensive care unit. He is then cared for by professionals who meet his physical needs but who may be unaware of his important emotional needs, or may be incapable of meeting them. A lung, heart, or kidney abnormality may preclude his being removed from the isolette for cuddling. A cleft lip or palate may prevent his sucking needs from being met. (He may need to be fed with a syringe. His elbows may have to be placed in restraints to prevent him from bending his arm to place his thumb in his mouth.)

How do parents usually react to extreme prematurity, defective organs, or severe illness in their newborn child? When there is a possibility that the child will not survive, they tend to hold themselves back from any emotional attachment to him. In a sense, they prepare themselves for his possible death by starting their "grief work" while he is alive. They may have a feeling of failure for having produced an imperfect child. They may have feelings of guilt for real or imagined reasons. For example, mothers who during pregnancy took medications that have been proven responsible for birth defects (e.g., thalidomide) feel personally responsible for what has happened.

Parents who have not been given a reason for a neonatal defect often look upon what has happened as a penalty. Women who have terminated previous pregnancies and men who have had extramarital affairs may look upon the child's deformity as punishment for what they now consider past misdeeds. Staff members can be of great help in reassuring parents that such actions were in no way responsible for the present problem. The parents may also need genetic counseling before another pregnancy is attempted, to determine whether subsequent pregnancies will have similar outcomes.

If the neonate survives, the parents usually start to become emotionally involved. Their interest in the baby is reawakened, and they attempt to assume the parent role. They become aware of the baby's special needs, and learn how to administer any special care. However, if future hospitalizations are needed, or surgery is anticipated, there may be continued interference with parenting. Fear of losing the baby continues until the problem is corrected or the baby dies.

When a baby dies, parents sometimes find that their outlets for expressing grief are limited. Hospital staff members are often too busy working out their own sense of failure about the death to help the parents. Staff members may try to "cheer up" the mother, but succeed only in isolating her further in her grief. Often husband and wife find it difficult to talk to each other about the death—each wants to protect the other from being wounded again. Staff members can be of greatest help when they acknowledge the death and encourage the parents to talk about it. Unreasonable guilt can often be examined and put to rest at this time, before it has a chance to cause major familial problems. The couple should be encouraged to talk to each other, regardless of the pain, because this helps each to ease his own burden while communicating on a more meaningful level with the other. The husband-wife relationship can be strengthened at this time if the staff does judicious counseling. Unless grief for the loss of this baby is worked through, future attempts at parenting with other children will be hampered.

Following successful delivery, usually the next crisis that occurs is weaning. This process, whether from bottle or breast, can be traumatic if it is done before the baby is ready for it, or if it is accomplished too quickly. If the baby's need to suck is not met adequately during feeding time because he is being weaned, he will have to find other ways of satisfying his oral drive. He may suck his thumb, fingers, tongue, lips, or pacifier. (At a later age, he may bite his fingernails as one reaction to the previous inadequate meeting of his oral needs.)

Those who work in postpartum areas can guide parents into an understanding of how weaning should be carried out. Many times, parents consider it a triumph when they succeed in weaning the child to a cup at an early age, regardless of the baby's need for more sucking. Knowledge about this infant need may help parents relax and let nature take its rightful course. The cup should be substituted for the bottle or the breast for only one feeding a day at the start. When the baby has adjusted to this, another feeding is changed. Progressively, as subsequent adjustments are made by the infant, the rest of the substitutions are made. The baby, not the parent, must set the pace. The baby may sense the approval or disapproval of the parents as he meets their goals.

A similar crisis often occurs during the time of toilet training. The eliminative process becomes the focus of family concern and possibly results in frustration for all. If the infant cannot let go of his urine or feces upon command, his actions may be interpreted by the parents as a sign of insolence or stubbornness. The lines of battle may be drawn for months or years, until the child has enough control over his own functions to perform on the toilet. Regression, with wetting or soiling by the child at a later date, may be met with anger. Enuresis (bed-wetting) or encopresis (soiling with feces) often causes severe problems within the household, for which parents may seek professional help. They often feel a sense of shame when the child continues to wet at night, and usually will not permit him to visit friends overnight, or go to sleepaway camp, for fear that others will discover their secret.

Children who continue to wet or soil themselves by school age may become targets of taunting by their schoolmates. Increased pressure by parents or others to remain dry and clean may have the opposite effect. The child becomes even less able to attain the parental goal set for him. Health workers can ease the situation by helping the parents to lessen the stresses of the child's daily living. They should emphasize the child's need for autonomy in as many areas as possible—including that of his excretory functions. The child's schoolteacher should also be advised of the problem, and should permit the child to go to the bathroom whenever he feels the urge to do so. In school, as at home, pressures should be eased as much as possible.

Starting school, in and of itself, constitutes a crisis. The child may rely on previously learned techniques of meeting new friends as he finds himself among strangers. If he has never had this opportunity before, he may have to experiment with ways to approach the teacher or other students. He may imitate his parents or remember a story or a television program which showed such meetings. If the child is outgoing (though not aggressive), is able to make himself understood, and is pleasant in his appearance and manner, he can usually fit in with the group. But what of the child whose speech is incomprehensible, or who has a noticeable physical defect, or who is overly passive or aggressive? He may find himself an outcast, not included in the activities of the others. A skilled teacher will help others accept the child, while also helping him to modify unacceptable behavior. Parents can be coaxed to include a new acquaintance in tempting family activities, and this may stimulate formation of a new friendship for their child.

Hospitalization of a young child, regardless of the reason for it, always creates a crisis situation. Separation from the family (particularly the mother) and the home can be very traumatic. A child's first reaction may be one of protest—he cries, screams, clings to his mother, even vomits. If the parent cannot remain with him, he may continue to cry until an overwhelming sense of despair sets in and he quiets down because he has given up. He develops a sense of detachment and is viewed as a "good" patient. He sits passively, doing whatever he is told, believing that he has been deserted by those whom he loved and trusted. Often hospital rules prevent parents from remaining with children because their presence "upsets" the *hospital* routine. Hospital personnel often ignore the fact that such a regulation upsets the *child's* routine. Workers who keep the whole child as the focus of their care will certainly encourage parents to remain with young children for as much of the time as possible, for they will recognize the need of the child to have the parent remain and the need of the parent to be with the child. Whenever possible, a parent should be permitted to sleep in the room with the child. If that is not possible, the visiting schedule should be flexible. Parents should be coached to tell the child when they are leaving, and when they will return. If the child cannot tell time, the parent should relate his return to hospital activity: "I will be back when you are eating breakfast." Placing a note to this effect at the bedside enables the staff to corroborate and reinforce the information for the child.

Beginning adolescence is another time when maturational crises occur. Growth patterns at this age, including the acquisition of secondary sexual characteristics, may disturb the individual's sense of identity. Neither child nor adult, the adolescent finds his goals changing, the demands upon him increasing. He must make many decisions for the future —whether to continue his education, what his vocational talents are, which friendships to continue, and how to withstand parental or peer pressures which do not coincide with his own desires. He wants complete autonomy on one hand, while continuing his dependency state on the other. He wants complete independence at times, but feels safer when parental limitations are set for him. Health workers can help parents accept this duality of behavior by explaining the need of the adolescent to try his wings while still within the security of the home.

If hospitalization takes place at this time, every effort should be made by the staff to provide as much autonomy for the patient as possible, within set limits. Insofar as is feasible, the adolescent should choose his own diet, determine his own care and the extent of his involvement with others, share a room with others in his age range, have appropriate activities available, be aware of limitations placed upon him, and be held to set limitations in all these areas.

Advance knowledge of sexual changes and drives should be available to both boys and girls. Unless menstruation has been discussed in advance, the first appearance of blood may be a fearsome episode for a girl. In the same way, his first nocturnal emission can be very upsetting to an unprepared boy. Health workers are frequently asked to present sex education programs to adolescents. Those who accept must be certain that the information they give is correct, and that the presentation itself encourages healthy attitudes towards sex and sexuality.

The older adolescent may leave home for college, and find himself once more in crisis. If he has been given the freedom to make his own decisions while at home, he will probably be less overwhelmed by all the responsibility which he must accept in this new situation. If he has always been told what to wear, what to eat, and what, where, and how to study, he may find decision-making very difficult. He may go wild with his new-found freedom, or be afraid to venture out of his room alone. Once more he is called upon to make friends among strangers. The individual whose early childhood attempts were successful may have no difficulties. If those early attempts were *not* successful, then he may be afraid of rejection and hesitate to involve himself with others. When youngsters' parents have provided them with opportunities to make decisions for themselves, the chances are that decision-making will not be a problem for the youth away from home. A youngster who is given the responsibility for choosing his own future at college, and is allowed to enroll in courses of his own choice rather than those selected by his parents, will have an easier time in establishing his own identity.

The high rate of suicide among college students is an indication of their inability to cope with the many problems that are present on the campus. Most college officials note keen competition among students for marks, particularly among those who plan to attend professional graduate schools. If the student finds the competition too strenuous, or feels that his parents are demanding too high a level of performance, severe depression may set in. He may decide to drop out of school "to find myself," or may turn to such avenues of escape as drugs, somatic complaints, homosexual or heterosexual love affairs, or the creation of a fantasy world. As a last resort, he may attempt suicide.

Crisis intervention centers are available on many campuses, manned by professionals or trained lay people, to provide an immediate outlet for students with emotions that are too difficult to handle alone. When such a center is not at hand, the personnel in the student health service may be called upon to provide emergency service. Workers must have the ability to listen without imposing their own values, while helping students to think their problems through.

Entering the job market is often another time of crisis. The availability of jobs for which the applicant has been prepared is a major factor in attaining a desirable position. Perhaps the market for one's skills no longer exists, and other types of work are unappealing. Then a feeling of worthlessness may set in. When a person's skills are very specific, and he cannot alter them, he may not be able to find any work that is satisfactory. The college-graduate applicant often finds that his superior education is no guarantee that he will be rewarded with a worthwhile job opportunity.

Selection of a job within one's area of competence may be made difficult by self-set standards. For example, the newly graduated chemical engineer may refuse to work for any company connected with products that are harmful to the environment, but if the only job that is available is in such a company, he may find it necessary to sacrifice his ideals.

Although satisfaction with one's work is important, that factor may have to be set aside for higher wages or a job more in line with one's abilities. Some people prefer to be in creative work but do not have the innate capabilities required for such jobs. They may have to accept less stimulating work in an administrative or secretarial capacity, and then they may feel frustrated by the lack of opportunity to be creative. If previous life experiences have encouraged creativity in hobbies or avocations, this need may be met. If, however, the person's creative talent has only been job-connected, the substitute situation will not provide any inner satisfaction. He then builds up tensions that may lead to accidents on the job, somatic complaints, or depression. This individual needs help in determining priorities—do the assets of the job situation outweigh the deficits, or should another job be sought?

Soon another crisis looms. Conventional marriage, although disregarded by many, still attracts a large number of couples. Reasons for marriage vary. The health worker who is present during the premarital physical is often able to pick up reasons why the contemplated marriage might not be a stable one. The prospective bride or groom may be using marriage to escape from an unpleasant home situation. Others may feel that this is their "last chance" for marriage. Still others may marry only to have children or to legitimatize them, or to be supported financially, or because "everybody else" is getting married. Premarital counseling in such instances may prevent a lifetime of unhappiness.

The next maturational crisis comes with pregnancy, which may be wanted, unwanted, planned, or unplanned. The wanted, planned pregnancy tends to be less upsetting than that which is not only unplanned but unwanted. The parents may blame each other in the latter case, and may vent their feelings on each other. They may feel trapped, and attempt to terminate the pregnancy. Even when such termination is done properly and legally, emotional problems about the right to end the life of another may ensue.

On the other hand, even the wanted, planned pregnancy leads to some emotional turmoil. The sudden realization by the parents that they will be primarily responsible for another human being, and that the responsibility is theirs around the clock, is often frightening. They may not have had role models available to learn how to be a parent and may worry about assuming this new role. Antepartum nurses have the opportunity to help prepare couples for parenthood. They should listen to what expectant mothers say or ask during their visits, and work with them to solve problems and overcome anxieties. This is as important as checking weights, blood pressures, and urines. If classes are given to prepare couples for childbirth, the nurse has the chance to watch husband-wife interactions. She is in a position to pick up unhealthy patterns, and to help the couple find acceptable ways of working out problems.

Husbands who have been prepared to help their wives through labor and delivery often describe the experience as "the most thrilling of my life." Wives feel a closeness to their husbands, and may comment, "I could not have done it without him." Yet even under these circumstances, mothers often speak about their feelings of unreality after delivery ("Is it really *my* baby? How could this have come out of me?") and the lack of a sense of motherliness. They are also usually beset by overwhelming fatigue, and may even have episodes of emotional lability, crying and laughing without control. Unless the postpartum nurse has explained the normality of such behavior in advance, the mother may suspect that she is "going crazy," and both husband and wife will worry about it unnecessarily.

Although crying episodes are normal after delivery, insomnia should arouse concern in the postpartum staff. Total lack of sleep may be the first sign of postpartum depression, and the patient should be watched closely for any other signs of depression. Immediate intervention is one way of preventing prolonged illness. The primiparous mother may be so overly concerned about her ability to care for both her newborn and her husband that she becomes immobilized. Multiparae worry about how the new child will fit into the established pattern of the household, and need reassurance that it is a solvable problem.

All too soon, the children have grown, and the "empty nest" syndrome becomes the scene of the next crisis. A woman who has spent her years "mothering," and has developed no outside interests, may suddenly feel unwanted and unneeded. Her reason for living is over—her task is finished. She has been so busy with her children that her relationship with her husband has disintegrated. To prevent this eventuality, women should be coaxed to develop outside interests *before* all the children leave. This can be done by health workers who prepare women for physical examinations, or who are present when women bring their children in for checkups. The importance of strengthening the husband-wife relationship should also be stressed throughout the years of child-rearing.

The times of menopause and the male climacteric may also be times of crisis. Self-doubts become prevalent as each partner realizes that the days of procreation are nearing an end. Retirement often coincides with this time, bringing a sense of failure because of unfulfilled dreams. If the individual has had a meaningful life, with a degree of success, the disappointments are usually limited. If, however, life has been a series of frustrations and compromises, it may be difficult to accept the fact that it is approaching the end. One may have to face old age without a mate, and with a narrowing circle of friends as people die. One's children move away, become busy with their own families and pursuits, so plans must be made for the elderly who live alone or for whom self-care is no longer feasible. As life nears its end, elderly people may regress to a state of childlike dependence, even when trying to maintain their own autonomy, just as they did in adolescence.

Health workers can encourage activities for the older person's physical status. They should be aware of community agencies which make such activities available, and which also provide the opportunity for new friendships. Physical problems must be considered, and arrangements made for securing proper medical attention. During the time when such care is given, the health worker should assess the patient's abilities and encourage him to live up to his physical and mental potential. The more active he is, the slower the aging process is likely to be, and the more satisfaction he is likely to derive from his life. In this way, he can *live* the later years of his life, and not simply deteriorate while just sitting and waiting for life to end.

PART TWO

Specific Approaches

The Anxious Patient

The feelings of tension, uneasiness, nervousness, and apprehension that are created by stress, the source of which may or may not be known to the patient or worker, are called anxiety.

Anxiety is one of the most common problems the health worker encounters in patients, whether they be at home, in a hospital, or elsewhere. It may become apparent through physical or behavioral symptoms which make the management of the patient difficult. This is particularly true when the worker either does not see the relationship of the patient's symptoms to his anxiety, or is unsure of how to handle the situation effectively. The worker himself may experience anxiety at such times.

Many factors contribute to the patient's anxiety. For example, think for a moment of the patient who is being admitted to the hospital. To the staff, this is a familiar routine—an everyday occurrence. To the patient, however, it may be a frightening experience, especially if he is unfamiliar with the hospital, its routine, and its personnel. He may be worried about the condition that brought him to the hospital, and concerned about such matters as how his family will manage in his absence, or whether his hospitalization will jeopardize his job. He may feel apprehensive about what will be happening to him minute by minute, day by day. Certainly, the patient who is confined to bed for long periods has plenty of time to dwell on himself and all the unknowns. He may, oftener than not, overhear bits of conversation or observe activities that he does not understand, and worry about their application to himself. He may experience a sense of helplessness, feel cut off, alone. The staff sometimes increases these feelings by trying to do everything for him and by describing the hospital rules and regulations as if the patient no longer had any right to make decisions about his own care. A busy staff may not take time to properly orient the newly admitted patient to the hospital or to his immediate environment.

The health worker himself may be functioning under pressure, causing his own level of anxiety to rise. He may be worried about getting all his tasks completed, especially when he has a large assignment. A heavy census, shortage of staff, and the energy required of that staff just to keep up with the daily activities of patient care, teaching, and administrative tasks, increase the worker's feeling that the last thing in the world he has time for is chatting with patients. Often he feels that a long, involved talk is not worth while, since it is unlikely to be productive. The worker may be even more anxious caring for a patient who is older than he is, or more intelligent, or more worldly.

Hospitalization is a threatening situation that may cause the patient to feel as though he is at the mercy of a vast impersonal institution. His physical being is placed in the care of others whom he may never have met before. The stresses he faces are many, and real, and he reacts to them with symptoms of anxiety—sweaty hands, tremors, rapid pulse, dilated pupils, diarrhea, or urinary frequency. Palpitations, restlessness, and indigestion are not uncommon. The patient may be tearful for no apparent reason, and may complain about everything and anything. The worker's efforts to please him are to no avail. He may regard whatever is said as a personal attack, and is easily angered. Or, conversely, he may act as though he is at a hotel for a few days' rest, laughing and joking with such consistent cheeriness that the worker reviews the chart, wondering if indeed the patient is in the right place. Because hospital nurses work so closely with patients, they are usually the first to note changes in patients' appearance, mood, and behavior. These changes may indicate that the patient is trying to relieve himself of inner feelings of tension which are mounting to the point of discomfort.

Patients often seek medical help for physically disabling symptoms, unaware that their symptoms are based on psychological factors. The patient does not realize that his symptoms have been provoked by emotional problems or situations, not by a physiological cause. Often only physical discomfort is felt; the patient is unconscious of the emotional cause.

Anxious patients are often regarded as difficult patients. This is because even extensive evaluation may not produce clinical evidence to explain the symptoms. One forty-year-old man was thought to have a rare disease. The necessary workup unfortunately caused him to dwell even more on his physical symptoms. The tests proved negative, but his symptoms continued to escalate. As a last resort, a psychiatric evaluation was requested. This revealed a host of complicated problems, such as his inability to separate emotionally from his parents, who were in the process of moving to another part of the country. In addition, he was very insecure about his position in the company for which he worked. His symptoms began to decrease as he became involved in regular psychotherapy.

The worker will do well to remember that every person, including himself, has moments of anxiety. The degree of anxiety determines whether it will be a constructive or destructive force. Mild to moderate anxiety helps a person to meet his life situations. Severe anxiety reduces that ability and inhibits the person from handling stressful situations. When anxiety begins to interfere with the patient's ability to cope with his many stresses, he uses symptoms and behaviors, such as those described above, in an attempt to relieve his intense feelings of discomfort.

THE APPROACH TO THE ANXIOUS PATIENT

Recognize the signs and symptoms of anxiety. Tremors, rapid speech, wringing of the hands, excessive perspiration, repetitious questioning, complaints of palpitation or rapid breathing, diarrhea, a feeling of knots in the abdomen, inability to focus attention on any one thing for a period of time, difficulty in concentrating or sleeping, continuous forgetfulness, frequent use of the call bell, are all signs of anxiety.

Don't assume that the patient's anxieties are totally due to his mental illness. One sixty-year-old gentleman refused heart surgery, believing that he would die during the procedure. His fear was that his death would enable his son, whom he disliked, to complete his college education by collecting on a large insurance policy in which he had been designated as the beneficiary.

Tolerate the patient's tenseness. All too often health workers seem more anxious to reassure themselves than their patients. If you find your own anxiety level rising, arrange for frequent relief periods by other staff members. This helps the patient to feel that he is not alone and that others —as well as you—are concerned and interested. At the same time, you will be able to function more comfortably and therapeutically when with him.

Do make an attempt to understand what triggers your own anxiety. One staff member was immobilized when assigned to care for a patient receiving an additional course of radiation therapy. The worker's own medical history revealed a previous mastectomy followed by radiation therapy. The parallels between her own illness and that of the patient increased her anxiety about her own condition to the point where she could not function therapeutically.

Be understanding of the patient's feelings. Let him know that you recognize his present state. Tell him, "You must be very uncomfortable now. But, as your condition improves you will feel more at ease." Don't involve him in loud, noisy, or complicated activities. Start with individual brief encounters which are firm but supportive. When the patient is able to cooperate, direct his energy into some productive and meaningful activity.

Do not make demands on the patient when his anxiety is high. Remember, he cannot cope with his situation as is, so one more stress may prove catastrophic.

Don't try to reassure the patient with empty explanations. "I'd be anxious too if my husband lost the bank book" or "Anyone would be anxious if they had parents like yours" are illustrative of statements that are usually ineffective because the patient doubts that anyone else would really have that same reaction. Additionally, if the patient thought he knew what was really causing his anxiety, he would have gained control of the situation long ago.

When approaching the patient, speak slowly, briefly, and concretely. This increases the likelihood that the patient will grasp what you say. Do not use meaningless phrases such as: "Just relax." "Don't be nervous." "There's nothing to worry about." "Control yourself." "I think you like to worry; it gives you something to do." "Just pull yourself together." "Some people are just natural born worriers."

Encourage the patient to verbalize his feelings about what he remembers that happened before he became anxious. If he doesn't remember, don't push. But every now and then gently lead him back to the subject. Soon he will remember situations and incidents that provoked his present responses and feelings. Help the patient to find healthier ways of responding to anxiety-producing factors. If he does not want to talk to you at a given moment, he may vehemently maintain that nothing is the matter and that you should mind your own business. Do not react as though he is doing something terrible by not wanting to bare his soul to you. Remember, you are there to help the patient and to meet his needs, not the reverse. Therefore, do not reject the patient by going off in a huff because he has rejected you. Say, "I understand that you may not feel like talking now, so I will come back in an hour when you may feel differently." And then do that; keep your word and return. This demonstrates to the patient that you really do care, are reliable, and that he can trust you.

Don't offer suggestions as to the possible causes of the patient's anxiety. Anxiety attacks are often triggered by unconscious factors. You may inadvertently focus on such a factor and thus increase his anxiety. Don't assume that you know what is worrying the patient. Remember that there is no substitute for direct questions when trying to obtain information from the patient.

Employ measures to increase the patient's comfort: Warm milk in the evening; no blaring radios; warm bath or shower; eliminate glaring lights.

Tell the patient you are concerned about him and his feelings. Let him know that by talking with him about those feelings and understanding them, you will be better able to understand and help him. Give him the opportunity to talk by saying, "I wonder how things have been going with you in general?" or, "It must be very difficult for you to be here, when your mind is on so many other things." The health worker who cheerfully grins and breezes into the room saying, "In a few hours you'll be fine" or "Everyone gets better on my floor" is hardly credible. It is far better to acknowledge the difficult time the patient is experiencing.

Do not dwell on what the patient is doing to relieve his tensions. He may be constantly calling for the nurse, persistently running up to the nurses' station, not taking medication, or otherwise ignoring the doctor's recommendations. Do not say, "Now, now, I expect much more from a person like you" or "You are acting like a two-year-old. Now grow up." Such remarks only reveal your anger and inability to change the situation.

Do not become defensive when the patient complains. He may not like the hospital food, his nursing care, or even the placement of his bed.

Instead, help him to talk about himself, to explain and describe to you what happened before he became upset.

Offer any reasonable explanations or information to clear up the patient's misconceptions about his condition. For example, the patient may erroneously believe that staff members are avoiding telling him about test results because he definitely has an incurable disease. Tell him, "The laboratory tests and reports have not yet been completed. There is nothing on the chart that states a definite diagnosis. Neither the doctor nor I know whether you have this disease. I can understand how difficult it must be to worry about this alone." These statements allow the patient to save face regarding his behavior, and at the same time encourage the realization that some of his worries may be unfounded.

Do not be surprised if logic is useless. The patient may see himself as physically ill, although this may not be so. This misconception can be corrected only at the rate tolerated by the individual. It is important to focus on the healthy and positive aspects of the way in which the patient functions rather than try to convince him that nothing is physically wrong.

Do not expect the patient to change his behavior immediately. Remember that the method he has chosen to make himself comfortable may be one that he has used to relieve anxiety throughout his life.

The Depressed Patient

Health workers are rightfully concerned about patients who show overt signs of depression. The patient who weeps easily and frequently or expresses thoughts of dying presents a problem to the staff. Before reaching this stage, he may have presented signs of mild depression that were not recognized as such—inability to concentrate, sleeplessness, poor appetite, constipation, amenorrhea, impotence, or disinterest in sex. He may have appeared unkempt and unshaven. He may have expressed thoughts of hopelessness, worthlessness, and even hinted at the possibility of suicide. Most of his thoughts were related to his loss of self-esteem. Motor activity impairment such as slowed speech and movement may have also been noted.

When a depression is recognized as such, the worker may want to intervene, but sometimes hesitates for fear that this will cause the situation to worsen. It is unlikely that he would be the *cause* of any further deterioration, since the reasons for the depression are probably deeply rooted, and unrelated to his actions. On the other hand, the fact that he shows interest, spends time with the patient, and listens to him is therapeutic in itself. It is important for the worker to let the patient decide how much, and when, he wishes to discuss any emotionally charged material.

Under certain circumstances, depression is a normal reaction. The individual who has lost a loved one, had a limb amputated, or been given a diagnosis of an incurable illness has the right to be depressed and to grieve. The patient will probably manifest decreased interest in his surroundings, boredom, and a tendency to ruminate about his loss. He cannot be expected to remain cheerful under such circumstances. As he adjusts to his new life situation, he comes to terms with himself, and the depression usually lifts. Health workers can help by listening to the patient as he talks, and by encouraging him to examine his feelings. This helps the patient free himself from his attachment to the lost individual and encourages him to seek new relationships.

The patient who cries, weeps, screams, or whines is expressing helplessness. His loss of control makes most staff members feel very uncomfortable. Yet tearfulness can be therapeutic in some situations. For example, a worker who remains with the patient and quietly says, "I understand how difficult this time is for you—crying sometimes helps us to deal with such situations," is letting the patient know that his crying is not frowned upon, and that he is not alone in his grief. As soon as he is able to control his tears, the worker should encourage him to verbalize his feelings about the specific problems that caused his weeping. It is not uncommon to discover that factors such as a lack of success in work, loneliness, concerns regarding physical appearance, or the feeling of a loss of masculinity or femininity have triggered the emotional reaction. When the worker understands what the patient's perception of the circumstances are, he can help him get his bearings and aid him in reorganizing his approach to life in a reasonably hopeful and realistic way.

The depression that is not based on external reality, or that becomes prolonged or incapacitating, requires a greater degree of intervention. For example, the worker would expect a patient to be relieved and happy when told, after a benign tumor has been removed, that no further treatment is needed. He would be concerned if the patient rejects this diagnosis, remains convinced that everyone is lying, and believes that he is going to die. At this point, the worker's efforts should be geared to helping the patient talk about his unhappiness. Possibly as they talk, they will uncover the situation underlying the patient's unhappy outlook, one which may be too much for the patient to face. Then more realistic thinking can be stimulated. At the same time the worker can encourage the patient to accept the current situation by repeating the facts about his condition, i.e., blood work normal, pathology report normal, recovery progressing satisfactorily.

Severe depression requires ongoing support of the patient by all staff members. The patient who is severely depressed has little desire or energy to do anything. Usually, he will not want to talk, or participate in any therapies because he thinks he cannot do them well and is fearful of exposing his weak points. Thus, his feelings of inadequacy and worthlessness increase. The worker, therefore, must assume the initiative in drawing the patient into conversation or activities. However, he should not expect the patient to be pleasant or grateful to him for this challenge to his behavior pattern. The patient may even express anger at the intervention. This, in effect, is a sign of improvement, for depression is largely the result of anger being turned inward upon oneself. Anger at another helps turn that feeling outward, and is less destructive to the patient.

Depressed patients often need a tremendous amount of care, approval, and attention. No amount of support ever seems adequate. Their level of sensitivity is so great that a comment such as "I'm unable to go to the gift shop for you now, but I will be free to do so later in the day" may be interpreted as a rejection. The patient's needs can never be completely satisfied and therefore he always feels cheated, frustrated, and unloved.

Often the behavior of the depressed person is very infantile. Family, friends, and professionals may become exhausted and angry when their efforts fail to bring about improvement in his condition. It is not unusual for those who are involved with the patient to withdraw and say, "I give up. No matter what I do, it isn't enough." This further increases the patient's feelings of rejection and worthlessness.

The patient who is depressed usually gets an initial bonus of sympathy, attention, and pity. However, the price that is paid for this secondary gain is draining, considering the lengths to which the patient must often go, such as abusing drugs or alcohol, attempting or threatening suicide, or denying himself any pleasurable moments. He may go to extremes to become the center of attention. In one instance, a young man took an overdose of drugs because he felt overshadowed by his sister at a family dinner party.

Every depressed patient has feelings of futility. Whether the patient says so or not, he has very likely felt like killing himself at some point. Often the health worker picks up these feelings in the course of conversation, perhaps after he has noticed that the patient looks particularly upset, and comments on this. Common utterances of the depressed patient are, "I wish I were dead," "If I had a bottle of pills I would take them," "My family can use my insurance," "I'll show him," "He'll be sorry." Such statements should be taken seriously. The health worker should confront the patient by asking what plan or method he will use to carry out his threat. Thinking, "Oh, he's just saying that; he'll never really do it," is dangerous wishful thinking. It is an excuse one gives one's self when unable to face the possibility of a successful suicide attempt.

In one instance, a patient told the health worker that she'd like to "end the whole thing." The busy health worker disregarded the remark and later that evening the patient took an overdose of pills that she had concealed from the staff on admission. In another situation, an alert health worker noticed a patient whom he knew to be depressed walking with a peculiar gait as she left the lunchroom. He followed her into her room and asked if anything was troubling her. As he spoke, the health worker showed genuine concern. As a result, the patient gave him a knife that she had concealed under the elastic waistband of her slacks. In another case, a patient told the health worker that she was planning to commit suicide at home. On discharge, she did just that.

The patient who is restless, paces, and is agitated presents symptoms that indicate the need for immediate intervention. He will often plead for help, saying, "I feel like jumping out of my skin" or "I feel like I'm going to explode." He should be closely watched to prevent any self-destructive actions. Medication is usually indicated to lessen his agitation.

The patient who contemplates suicide is desperate. His judgment and thinking are impaired because of his depressed emotional state. Therefore, every precaution should be taken to protect him from his inability to control himself. It goes without saying that the physician and the on-coming shift must be alerted about the patient's statements and thoughts.

THE APPROACH TO THE DEPRESSED PATIENT

Initiate the approach. "You look unhappy today. Perhaps it will help if we talk about what's troubling you." Be alert to the suicide potential of patients who demonstrate lower levels of self-interest and who make suicidal statements.

Help the patient tolerate his illness until he can see and feel the situation differently. When the patient talks about suicide, the health worker should emphasize his concern for the patient, while letting him know that the staff can take over and protect him until he feels better. He can say, "I believe that you feel very unhappy now. People often feel that way when they are ill and need protection, temporarily, from themselves. The staff and I will not let you harm yourself, but will protect you until you have recovered sufficiently." Proceed to take any precautions deemed necessary.

Tell the patient that you understand and recognize his feelings. Tell him you have known others who have felt the same way at times. You can say, "When a situation like this arises, people often feel helpless before they have had the opportunity to think it through."

Let the patient know that you feel he is worthy. Note his participation in activities. "You certainly are helping us by filing those cards." However, don't overdo the flattery, because excess praise often reinforces the patient's feelings that because he is really worthless you are trying to make him feel good.

Show the patient you care about him. Stay with him, accept his silences, and tolerate his tears. Be nonjudgmental. Accept him at his present level.

Discourage the depressed patient from making major decisions. He may think of selling his house, making a new will, buying or selling stock, obtaining a divorce. Get him to delay such actions.

Pay attention to the patient's daily hygiene. Offer assistance and direction when necessary. Keep him from appearing unkempt because he doesn't have the strength to brush his hair, shave, or change his clothes. Be patient and controlled with the patient when he behaves so helplessly. Be aware of your own frustration and avoid ignoring or rejecting him, since this would only increase his feelings of worthlessness.

Help the patient to reorganize his capabilities and attitudes in a hopeful, realistic light as he improves. Offer him hope by communicating your belief that changes can be made, and that alternate solutions for his problems can be found.

Plan activities according to the patient's degree of depression and the place in which he is being treated. Active participation in sports, when feasible, is a helpful way of working out feelings of aggression. Tasks should be simple, and not require concentration; for example:

1. In the home: polishing furniture, folding laundry, scrubbing vegetables.

2. In the general hospital: setting up new charts, copying notices for the nursing staff, watering plants.

3. In the psychiatric hospital: recreational therapy (handicrafts, dancing, painting, poetry); occupational therapy (woodwork, sandpapering furniture, typing); classes in art or poetry. Individual and group therapy are also important factors in treatment.

Allow the patient plenty of time to react to your approach and to respond.

The Helpless Patient

Many patients coming into a psychiatric hospital have lost all sense of self-worth. Incapacitated by illness, they have become unable to function effectively in any area of living. Some have lost jobs and/or been unable to maintain their former positions, and may have been replaced in their family or community roles. Constant worry about not being successful increases the fear of failure, and causes the person to avoid acceptance of any new responsibility or taking part in any new ventures. If the patient does not assert himself in social, sexual, or work areas, he avoids the possibility of further loss of approval.

The patient's helplessness severely restricts his life. Often he is a prisoner in his own home, refusing to go anywhere unless accompanied by someone. Characteristically, he appears depressed, has a pessimistic attitude with little self-confidence, and exhibits anxiety in any situation where he feels alone or is away from a safe environment such as his home.

The helpless patient commonly complains of extreme fatigue which rest does not alleviate. His fatigue is usually greater in the morning, presumably after a good night's sleep. Conversely, he usually feels better and has more energy at night.

Helplessness is caused by a combination of early experience, anticipation of future events, and present circumstances. The health worker needs to evaluate factors in the patient's environment that may be influencing his behavior. For instance, a forty-five-year-old woman, reluctant to separate from her college-bound daughter, concealed her feelings by developing physical symptoms which left her bedridden and helpless. This resulted in a cancellation of the daughter's plans to live at school. Each time the youngster attempted to leave home, the mother's symptoms escalated markedly. This changed only after the mother was actively engaged in long-term therapy.

Well-meaning attempts by the health worker to encourage the patient to help himself are often resisted. Activities are shunned. The patient cannot even take care of his own daily routine. He never seems to know what to do, constantly flounders, and is unable to make even the simplest decisions for himself. He denies any part of the responsibility for his situation, and blames all his difficulties on other people or factors beyond his control. This behavior is reminiscent of that exhibited by a small child. In essence, the patient *has* regressed emotionally to his childhood years and is using old patterns of behavior in seeking gratification for his physical and emotional needs. It is as though he is saying, "Take care of me because you can see I just can't do it myself."

The patient's helplessness, his inability to do for himself, to make such simple decisions as what to wear, what to do right now, what to order from the menu, what to read, or how to take the next step, tend to evoke feelings of deep sympathy. The worker feels inclined to do for the patient what he is unable to do for himself. This may satisfy the worker's need to be helpful and needed, but increases the patient's helplessness by reinforcing his need to be dependent on others. Through all this, the worker may even neglect other patients who, on first impression, seem to need him less. Those others may then harbor ill feelings against the worker and even greater resentment against the patient who is taking up so much of his time.

The helpless patient avoids taking responsibility for himself or others. In this way, he cannot make a mistake, and thus is protected from being blamed by others. He withdraws from the world around him; friendships are lost, and family relationships are barely sustained.

Over a period of time, the patient's continued helplessness may evoke anger and a sense of frustration in those caring for him. They may begin to resent his inability or unwillingness to communicate, which prevents him from gaining any insight into his basic difficulties. When staff members begin to feel the weight of his helplessness, or assume that the patient just cannot be helped or does not appreciate all their efforts in his behalf, they may begin to ignore him. This justifies the patient's self-evaluation of being an unworthy and unlikable person. He says to himself, "Why try when no one cares?" Helplessness is a defense used by patients who generally feel that they have no worth. Unfortunately, the use of helplessness does not solve their problems, but instead, prevents meaningful interaction with others from taking place. It also stifles any growth toward a healthier behavior pattern.

THE APPROACH TO THE HELPLESS PATIENT

Use a kind but firm approach to reach the patient whose fears have immobilized him. A gentle but positive tone of voice and short, clear sentences will let the patient know that the worker recognizes the helplessness, but does not feel the situation is hopeless. The worker can say, "You feel as though you are not able to care for yourself at this time. That will change as you begin to feel better." This implies that the situation is temporary, and leaves the future open for improvement. The helpless patient needs patience and support while he learns to care for himself. The worker should focus on such simple tasks as grooming, care of one's room, and selection of food at meal-time.

Direct the patient's attention to his small gains or successes in activities instead of stressing his shortcomings. This increases his sense of accomplishment and, at the same time, supports his positive feelings about himself. For example, the worker can say, "Today you were able to finish making your bed and attend a group meeting."

Deal with the present when you talk with the patient. Focusing on the here and now counteracts his feelings of helplessness that arise from his inability to discuss the past.

Encourage a positive relationship with the patient so that he will enter into a discussion about himself. Clues to the patient's helplessness may appear as he talks of events in his childhood. Frequently the history reveals the presence of a parent who stifled any initiative or outward expression of feelings.

Enlist the patient's cooperation in planning his treatment, self-care, and therapeutic activities. This will increase his sense of control, and strengthen his defenses. If the patient functioned at all prior to his illness, direct his attention to those areas and stress his accomplishments—working at a job, cleaning the house, preparing meals, doing volunteer work, driving a car, meeting social obligations.

Allow plenty of time for the patient to complete a task. Help him see that errors are correctable, and need not be dwelt upon. The helpless patient's fear of making mistakes usually goes back to his childhood handling by critical parents. Such a patient has learned to avoid criticism by giving up in the face of difficulty. Stress the importance of the "doing," rather than perfection.

Encourage any attempt by the patient to assume responsibility for himself or others; e.g., setting up the room for a planned activity, erasing the blackboard, baking a cake, stamping charts.

Help the patient to experience success in a trying situation. Point out his positive efforts towards self-help, e.g., his ability to remain with the group for a full hour, to talk with the therapist or to relate to other people at mealtime, and his improved appearance.

The Grieving Patient

The grieving individual displays a steady, continuous affect of sadness. He cries, has difficulty falling asleep, and eats little. Usually, he complains of weariness, although he has strength enough to manage himself. He is anxious, and his memory may be poor. His feeling of being dependent and needing people to help him increases. Sometimes such patients become clinging, almost helpless. However, most grieving patients are well oriented and in good contact with reality. Their self-esteem may not be threatened or appreciably compromised.

Grief is usually due to a loss the patient has sustained in the past, or one that he presently anticipates. People grieve for various kinds of losses —a very dearly loved person; a material thing such as a boat, house, diamond ring; or even for an opportunity which has passed one by.

Grief that results from loss usually subsides gradually. Sometimes, however, a person's reaction to his loss does not subside and he needs to be hospitalized. This does not mean that he is not grieving. He is! But because of preexisting conflicts and difficulties he isn't able to handle his grief. The new situation uncovers other problem areas that had previously been dormant. The health worker should be aware that anyone with unresolved difficulties may have a grief reaction that can result in a potentially serious depression.

People who have a normal response to grief do not require hospitalization. Their extreme distress abates within a reasonable time period (usually about six weeks). They adjust to their loss, and do not blame themselves for that which could not be prevented. Friends and family help by allowing them to talk about their feelings without feeling ashamed or humiliated. When a person is unable to function because he cannot accept the loss, and continues to dwell on it while berating and condemning himself, psychiatric treatment is probably needed. Such a reaction to a permanent, irretrievable loss is illustrated by the following cases: a girl whose lesbian partner deserted her for someone else was beset by a constant feeling of sadness and inability to concentrate on her college courses; a woman whose child died from leukemia was unable to have satisfactory sexual relations with her husband; a woman whose dog was killed by a car cried openly for weeks.

Anticipated losses may also trigger a grief response. Examples of mourning for losses in advance include the college-bound adolescent anticipating the loss of family life; the woman whose husband is drafted anticipating changes in her life pattern; the man transferred to a new job fearing the loss of old friends.

A loss usually involves someone or something that has a special meaning or significance for the loser. Without the loved object he feels he will be less capable, less able to function, and less happy. He may interpret the loss as a rejection and worry that he will also be rejected by other meaningful people in his life. The individual experiences feelings of guilt. For instance, one woman whose spouse died felt that she had not been warm and loving enough during their life together, and now it was too late; she began to experience deep remorse. Another patient expressed the feeling of not having done enough to help care for his wife during her lingering illness. Still another patient experienced moderate grief but had intense guilt feelings when his wife died from multiple sclerosis in a nursing home; he felt that his placing her there contributed to her death.

Some individuals verbalize their anger in their grief. A college student related that his father's death meant that he no longer could continue attending an elite university. His important plans for the future were now interrupted, and he was angry.

In normal grieving, the person does not blame himself for the loss. Although there is the feeling of being lost or empty, the person's self-esteem is not lowered. His grief can usually be worked through with help from friends and family who support him and provide the opportunity for him to express feelings in regard to the loss.

Some individuals show very little overt reaction to the loss at the actual time it occurs, demonstrating an avoidance of emotional discomfort. Instead, they may continue well until an apparently minor incident appears to trigger the grief reaction. One patient accepted her twenty-three-year-old daughter's death from leukemia and returned to work almost immediately, functioning well for over a year. Then her talkative parakeet died and she became tearful, began ruminating over her loss, and complained of weariness to the point where she could no longer continue in her job. In another case, a man whose son was killed in a car accident continued seemingly well until six months later when his car (which had previously belonged to his son) broke down and needed extensive repairs. He became morose, irritable, and wept openly that life would never be the same again.

The length of grieving, the intensity of the symptoms, the degree of disturbing thoughts, the relevance of behavior (reality contact), the pressure of delusions, and the extent to which the individual's living is diminished in proportion to the particular loss involved, help the worker to make some conceptual distinction between neurotic depression (a reactive grief) and psychotic depression. For example, an elderly man who lost his wife following a lengthy illness became quite sad and stopped taking part in the many activities they had previously participated in jointly. For a while all he could think about was his wife and the happy times they shared together. He cried a great deal and complained of insomnia and fatigue. This continued for two months when a close friend insisted that he see a doctor. The doctor advised hospitalization. In the therapeutic environment, the patient began to accept his loss. He began to interact with others on the unit who had had similar experiences, and were working on ways of dealing with their difficulties. He found he was able to concentrate when staff distracted him from his loss. Suicidal thoughts related to his loss of hope diminished. His self-esteem increased as the void in his life was replaced with renewed interest in old hobbies and new interest in group activities. Gradually his grief was relieved, and he returned to normal.

If a patient's grief is prolonged, he may begin to idealize the deceased in order to deny the negative aspects of the relationship. For example, a forty-five-year-old patient who had lost her husband five years earlier claimed that he was the most fantastic, kind, brilliant, caring man in the world. No one could ever be as good a provider, as devoted a husband and father. After many weeks in group therapy, she identified with the angry feelings expressed by another participant who spoke of her husband's authoritarianism and inflexibility. The patient began to recognize her own feelings of having felt stifled during her marriage, as well as her failure to assert herself when it came to making decisions or disciplining her children. Her reliance on her husband, and her passivity, kept peace in the household. As she expressed her previously suppressed anger, her need to deny her feelings and the glorification of her spouse lessened considerably.

When grief is prolonged (as in a reactive depression) the individual continues to dwell on the loss, experiences guilt, and condemns himself for what has happened. His suffering becomes abnormal and, if not treated, may progress to a deep depression. (See "The Depressed Patient," p. 65.)

Although a loss may be accepted, the adjustments, disruptions, and changes in other aspects of a person's life may prove to be overwhelming when superimposed on the initial trauma. Such was the case of the patient whose husband was drafted into service. She dealt with the separation fairly well, but the subsequent loss of social relationships because married friends no longer extended invitations to "singles" and the financial hardship due to the husband's lower income as an army employee were additional stresses that she responded to with grief. In another case, a very competent woman learned that her husband was going to leave her for a woman older than herself. She blamed herself for not doing enough to hold the marriage together. Besides the loss of her husband, she had to face a disturbing legal procedure. Her previously stable household seemed devastated, and the care of her children without their father just too much. She became grief-ridden and dwelt on the loss of her past happiness. Both of the cases cited here involved the effects of harsh and sudden changes in circumstances that caused a reactive depression (grief) which was neither neurotic nor psychotic.

The grief reaction of a person who experiences a loss will vary according to how he interprets the loss. This is usually dependent on the depth and quality of the relationship involved and his past experiences and associations with the lost object or relationship. For example, a patient who had felt deserted by her parents when she was hospitalized for several years as a small child, reacted with uncontrollable grief when they moved to another state, although she was by this time a seemingly well-adjusted adult. She interpreted her parents' move as another desertion, and relived the intense trauma of her childhood.

Similarly, a twenty-year-old woman was immobilized by grief after her lover ended their two-year relationship. This rejection rekindled memories of her parents' divorce and her father's remarriage and relocation to another state when she was sixteen years old. Her grief was, in fact, based on the earlier incident, which she had never resolved.

One factor which may influence grief reactions is the degree to which the person anticipated or prepared for the loss. Another factor is the extent of trust the person has in his ability to survive alone. Steps taken to assure continuity for the survivor are important. For example, a woman whose spouse was terminally ill with cancer spent the year preceding his death becoming acquainted with all their legal and financial affairs. She enlisted his help in learning how to manage their situation. In addition, she enrolled in a secretarial review course. When her spouse died, she grieved, but the knowledge that she could continue on her own did much to prevent her grief from becoming destructive.

Similarly, all patients who enter the hospital experience a sense of loss. Hospitalization is a stressful period since it entails separation from family and friends, loss of one's normal roles, loss of a familiar and comfortable environment, and possibly loss of income or savings. The patient who recognizes that the separation or loss is only temporary is able to find comfort in the knowledge that he will recover. Get well cards, calls, and visits from friends also help to reassure the patient that he has not really been deserted. Thus his self-esteem is not appreciably decreased and his reaction is minimal, with little real discomfort. For example, one patient may react by complaining of inability to obtain adequate rest at night. Still another may complain of rumbling in his stomach and of not being able to eat as well as usual. Both complaints can be related to the patient's stress during his period of hospitalization.

THE APPROACH TO THE GRIEVING PATIENT

Provide and encourage an opportunity for the patient to discuss his feelings. When the patient talks about his loss, accept his remarks. As he talks, the intensity of his feelings will diminish, and it will be possible to distract him by introducing other subjects. Do not tell the patient to "dry your eyes" or say, "Come on now; big boys don't cry"; or "You'll only make yourself sicker by carrying on this way." Such statements reinforce the patient's sense of helplessness (the feeling that he cannot help himself). Encourage the patient to join a community group which helps the bereaved.

See that the patient avoids stimulating group activities during the evening. The grieving patient often has difficulty sleeping, and any excitement on the unit should be stopped before bedtime. Keep the patient on a schedule, e.g., breakfast, rest, activity, lunch, rest, occupational therapy, rest, and so on. Restrict his daytime sleeping by introducing activities that keep him awake. Encourage him to stay up during the early evening so he will be sleepy when bedtime comes. A warm shower or bath as well as sleeping medication a half hour before bedtime are helpful in inducing sleep.

If the patient wants to overeat, do not dwell on it. Acknowledge his hunger but tell him that eating won't solve his problem. Offer food, nicely prepared, but in small amounts.

Facilitate eye contact by sitting where the patient can see you. Although he may be unable to respond initially, remember that he still needs attention. The worker must initiate the approach. The person feels lost, isolated, and as though he is carrying a burden. He is unable to ask for help. Interrupt his preoccupation by directing him towards former interests. Support his endeavors. Don't rush him or insist that he answer you.

Supervise the patient's physical care. Gently correct his bathing or mouth care habits; his table manners. Avoid harshness. Remember that maintaining a good physical appearance often influences one's mood. Influence the patient to use the hospital beautician or barber, if one is available.

Help the patient to confine his thinking to the here and now. Do not talk about the future because he is unable to see that far. Help the patient identify his present feelings in relation to his loss, i.e., his denial, anger, bewilderment. Show the patient that these feelings are common in people who have suffered a loss. He can accept his feelings about his illness better if you allow him to talk about them openly.

Help the patient alleviate his guilt or an overzealous conscience. Let the patient discuss the extent of his suffering in light of what he feels he omitted to do in the past. The worker might say, "You were not able to drive your friend through the snowstorm because your employer specifically requested you not to leave the office at that time. I can recognize your feelings that resulted from his subsequent fatal accident as he drove to the airport. But isn't it time to call a truce with yourself? You certainly have suffered so much already" or "If your friend were here, what suggestion do you think he would have for you at this time?"

Accept the patient's tears. Halting tears is not necessarily an objective, but if the patient is able to stop his crying, it may be reassuring to him to realize that he has regained a measure of self-control. Ask him to look directly at you, and talk with him.

Try to settle incidents that make the patient angry at the time they occur. If the patient seems angry about not speaking to the doctor, not getting a telephone call he expected, or missing snack time, talk with him about it and try to correct the difficulty immediately so that the patient won't brood about it later.

Do not be judgmental or rejecting. Do not view the patient as uncooperative if he is slow to accept his loss. This takes time. But the worker should be aware of when it happens because mobilization of what is left occurs only after a loss has been accepted.

Be aware that although grief is normal, it can become an illness if prolonged over four to eight weeks.

Express interest in the patients as physical beings. Interest is shown by asking when they last showered or applied makeup, how they slept last night, and whether or what they ate. This helps patients feel cared for and enhances their self-esteem.

It is not uncommon for the grief-stricken patient to become angry and blame the health professional for his loss. Do not become defensive. Accept the patient's irritability, while pointing out reality, injecting doubt into the validity of his claims. "Your wife lived for ten years as a result of medical treatment for her tumor. It sounds like she received quite a bit of medical help."

Encourage ventilation of the person's feelings regarding the loss and his life with the lost person. Most of the time, others (family, friends) have stifled any expression of feelings.

Keep in mind that the bereaved person faces changes in his life. He may have to assume additional responsibilities and reevaluate his resources, work, residence, social life, leisure time, and status. These are real problems which add to the patient's misfortune.

The Hallucinating Patient

Hallucinations are episodes in which the patient hears, sees, smells, tastes, or feels what does not exist in reality. In other words, his perceptions do not have any outside stimulus, but come from inside himself.

Hallucinations may be associated with many conditions. Contributing factors include: surgery; disturbance in the body's electrolyte balance; head trauma; severe metabolic changes; brain tumor; aging; respiratory conditions; severe psychic stress (psychosis); drug reaction; alcoholism. Another cause may be prolonged isolation, during which the patient is alone a great deal of the time and, as a result, suffers from a lack of stimulation to his sensory motor system.

The worker can pick up obvious clues that will let him know the patient is hallucinating. He may notice the patient staring into space intently and paying no attention to the immediate environment or to any activity occurring nearby. The worker's attempts at communication are rebuffed. The patient may appear terribly frightened and report that snakes or devils or saints are surrounding him, or that a deceased parent or child had been with him. Or he may sit quietly, seemingly untroubled. The patient appears preoccupied and doesn't participate or cooperate with his daily care and treatment. These nonexistent images demand all of the patient's attention.

The worker does not know what the patient "sees" unless he asks. This should be done in a tone of voice that is of sufficient volume and clarity to catch or hold the patient's attention. For instance, a staff member may say, "Mr. Simpson, I am Mrs. Best. What are you looking at?" or "Tell me, what do you see now?" It is important to use the patient's name in addressing him, since most patients will respond to their names. This identification reinforces, for the patient, who he is, even if he has forgotten who or where he is, and identification of the worker helps the patient reenter reality with a minimum of embarrassment. A patient may readily respond to such intervention with, "My aunt was here"; "Daggers are pointing at me"; "The rocks are ready to roll down the mountain." If so, the worker can deal with the patient's experience, and at the same time can note that he himself has not seen or heard what the patient is describing.

Generally, it is not useful to question the reality of a hallucinating experience too soon, since such a challenge may increase the patient's anxiety to the point of making him unreachable. He may then deny what is happening. For example, one patient was observed talking to "the nice little bugs" and was counting, "One, two, three." When asked about this, she denied the entire experience, even though she appeared very bewildered as to where she was and what was happening to her.

The health worker can show his appreciation of the patient's reluctance to share his experience and of his anxiety when the issue is pursued, by saying, "Sometimes people have the unique experience of thinking they see objects or people, or that they hear sounds. This is usually just a part of the person's illness and disappears gradually as he improves." Such a statement offers reassurance while letting the patient know that the nurse understands and is concerned.

In certain instances, usually when the patient is quite ill, staff members may be incorrectly identified as the patient's beloved mother, old friend, teacher, aunt, or sister. At other times, the worker or any one else in the area may be seen as a hated, mean, hostile person who is out to "get" the patient. Voices, smells, or sounds may heighten the patient's misidentification. An eighteen-year-old psychotic girl responded to the health worker's voice by referring to him as her "teacher" and said, "You always loved me. I love you. You taught me photography. Can I go to school now?" She then accused the doctor, who smoked the same brand of cigarettes that her father had smoked, of being her "rotten father." "You always tell me you hate me and that I'm bad and nothing but trouble. Don't touch me."

It is easy to discover the patient who is having auditory hallucinations, for he will be observed talking with an unseen entity to whom he is attentive and responsive as though listening for answers. The ongoing conversation may last for seconds, minutes, or longer. On occasion, the quietly attentive worker may find himself involved in the hallucinatory experience. For example, the patient may turn to him and say, "Hear how he talks to me. He said he is going to kill me. You heard him." Again, the worker makes clear to the patient that the voice has not been audible to others.

Auditory and visual hallucinations may occur together. One middle-aged woman insisted that the problem that most interfered with her life was not the fact that she lived with her mother, with whom she had shared the care of an aged grandmother for the past seventeen years, but rather that she was involved in continual conversations with different men whom she said appeared on the walls of her room and exhausted her to the point where she was no longer able to eat or sleep. She said they had even pursued her to the hospital, where they continued to insist that she talk with them. The patient admitted that she knew others did not see or hear these men, but that they still bothered her terribly. Obviously, these hallucinations were filling a void that she had felt keenly during her many years of loneliness.

On admission, the patient usually responds honestly to routine questions as to whether hearing voices or seeing things have been a problem. Sometimes the worker has been informed of the problem beforehand by a relative who has accompanied the patient. If so, he can state openly, "Your mother mentioned that the voices you hear interfere with your ability to concentrate at home or at work and with your ability to get along with people. Is this so?" This gives the patient an opportunity to talk about the problem further. If he has already denied having hallucinations, the relatives' report can be used to probe the subject but this must be done gently so that the patient doesn't feel threatened.

Workers should report the hallucinations, with descriptive details, to other involved staff members, noting any events that may be contributing factors. Sharing this information helps to uncover the basis for the hallucinations. Discussion of how you managed the patient successfully encourages consistent treatment. It also helps to lessen the anxiety of workers who fear being with a patient whose behavior is "crazy."

As the worker pursues the details of the patient's hallucinatory experience, he must remain aware that the patient feels the experience deeply. He is usually convinced of its reality and is influenced by it. Because of this, the more information the worker has about the experience, the more effective and clearly defined his interaction will be. He must discover what the voices tell the patient, what the visions are, and what may precipitate the experience and/or influence its frequency.

THE APPROACH TO THE HALLUCINATING PATIENT

If you suspect that a patient is hallucinating, use open-ended questions that require more than a "yes" or "no" answer. For example, "What did you decide to do this afternoon?" may elicit a response such as, "I'm going with this policeman to court." This is more informative about the patient's state than asking, "Are you all right?" to which the patient can respond, "Yes." In this instance, there was no policeman, nor was the patient going to court.

 As you approach the patient, state who you are and what your role is. Say, "Tell me about your day today" or "What's happening today?" Sit next to the patient, or walk along beside him. Your availability will make him feel your interest, warmth, genuine concern, and desire to talk with him. Spending time with the patient will enable you to more easily assess what is really happening. Reply to his lucid comments about his surroundings, his clothes, or his family. These are real. Be kind but firm when you refer to what the patient states he alone has seen or heard. Always let him know—outright or by implication—that you believe what he states but, for example, that you do not hear the voice he speaks of. This can be implied by asking, "Is the voice you hear male or female?" "Does the vision you see remind you of anyone or anything from your past?" Arguing with the patient and trying to convince him that his perception is unreal is futile. It only increases his anxiety and his use of denial, which stifles further communication. Ask the patient to describe his experience. "What do the voices say?" "What do you see?" "What is your reaction to what you smell?"

 Maintain adequate protection and surveillance for the patient. This is a must for one who is frightened and/or appears to be responding to commands that he may think are telling him to run, jump, or hurt himself or others. The patient may have to be moved to a padded room on a closed unit so that he will not harm himself or others. A nurse may have to remain with him for extended periods of time in order to help him cope with his experience and interrupt it, if possible. Keep the patient's environment familiar whenever feasible, so that he does not have to readjust to the physical setup. Don't allow him to be flooded with visitors and well-meaning friends. Too much stimulation may increase his confusion.

Always try to use a verbal response. Arm gestures, finger-shaking, showing approval or disapproval by head movements or grimacing are ambiguous and may intensify the patient's hallucination. Use clear, uncomplicated responses when answering his questions. Try to orient him to time, place, and activities each time you approach him.

Try to get the patient to focus his interest on what is real or happening at the moment. "What kinds of flowers are in that vase?" "Who brought them to you?" "What is the book on your table about?" "What kinds of stories do you enjoy reading?" "What activities do you like?" "Was your dressing changed today?" "Did you notice any drainage on it?" "Was the bath water warm enough?" "What kind of a day are you having today?" Always present reality when responding to an hallucinating patient. For example, "You say bats are flying. I do not see any. You are safe."

As the patient begins to improve, include him in group activities in which only a few members participate. The focus should be on "doing," as in occupational therapy—painting, sanding, woodworking, making ceramic objects, or sewing, for example. Encourage the patient to go on outside walks when this is possible and to participate in dancing, exercise classes, bingo, card playing, games, baking, or other available activities. Your joining in these activities will encourage the patient to accept them as valuable. Activities keep the patient focused on reality, reduce his level of tension, provide satisfaction and gratification, and expose him to interactions with others. When the patient is able, group or individual discussions that focus on preparing him for living in the community should be stressed. Discussions may center on such items as transportation, selection of proper clothing, how to obtain a job or gain admission to a school, budgeting, or how to improve existing skills. Encourage the patient to participate in his own care to the degree that he is able. Help him with what he is unable to do.

Always treat the patient with consideration, respect, and a concerned attitude. A warm human response will have a substantial beneficial effect, even though the patient may appear to be unaware of what is happening.

The Rejecting Patient

The rejecting patient says over and over again: "No"; "I don't want to"; "Not now"; "What for?"; "It's dumb." He refuses what staff members may offer, whether it is a back rub, a walk, a drink of juice, or whatever. He usually does not take part in scheduled activities. When he does attend he does not participate but complains throughout that the therapy is useless. He may then say that he is sitting in only because he has been coerced into it, or because he wants to please his family, or that attending is the road that leads to discharge because his cooperation will be noted in the nurses' report. All efforts to talk with the patient are futile. The worker becomes aware of doing all the talking in order to keep up the facade of a conversation. The patient shows little response. When he anticipates that the worker is on the verge of saying something to him or coming his way to make a request, he may protest animatedly either in gestures or speech. In other words, the patient shuts the staff out by closing the door on any help that is offered. He does not see that it is his behavior that prevents others from working with him. His misinterpretation gives rise to an inner feeling that nothing will ever help—that he can never recover.

No one wants to feel rejected, refused, shut out, hurt. Yet this is just how the rejecting patient anticipates he will feel if he becomes involved. In order to prevent this, he avoids *any* involvement. He scorns help, avoids interaction, says: "No; leave me alone"; "Please go away"; "I don't want to"; "That's that, I've had it"; "Please stop bothering me"; "I don't need your help"; "You're a big pest." What the worker must understand is that these patients have usually had more than their share of rejection. They feel worthless, and are asking for proof of staff interest in them. Some have experienced the early loss of one or both parents and were consequently shuffled from home to home. Others have come from broken homes in which neither parent wanted them. Early socioeconomic difficulties may have caused much deprivation. Some patients may have had parents who were so busy with social or work activities aimed at achieving status and position for themselves that they did not realize that more than food and clothing are needed for the healthy emotional growth of children. Or they may have been cold, stern people who never gave their affection freely; if love was given, it was offered as though it were a chore or an obligation. A rejecting patient may have been hospitalized during his early life because of physical illness, abandonment, or antisocial behavior. As a result, he may have experienced actual physical and emotional isolation from any kind of familiar environment or close relationships.

The feeling of being unwanted and unloved may be deeply rooted or the patient's early history may reveal no actual episode of rejection. Sometimes there is a symbolic episode which has been misinterpreted by the patient as a rejection. In one case, a twenty-year-old girl spoke of her resentment when her younger sister was born almost fifteen years before. She interpreted the birth as a sign that her parents no longer loved or wanted her, that they were rejecting her. In another case, a thirty-year-old female who had received financial help from her sister-in-law expressed profound feelings of rejection when the same sister-in-law also provided help to another family member. It takes a long time for the rejecting patient to begin to place trust in others or to feel even a little bit good about himself. The initial effort often has to be made by the worker, in order to make the patient realize that at least one person thinks he has worth. One rejecting patient repeatedly refused to come out of her room, eat with others, or talk with anyone. Her response to the nurse's concern was, "Who would be interested in me? I've never amounted to anything and never will." She appeared stunned when the nurse proceeded to bring two lunch trays into the room, and sat down to eat with her. However, this initiated a meaningful relationship between them.

Sometimes a person is promised something that he really counts on and if the promise is not fulfilled, he interprets this as a rejection of himself, even though the explanation offered refutes the thought. One extreme example of this occurred when a patient's husband, having promised her a trip after he retired, died suddenly three days before his retirement, thereby making it impossible to fulfill his promise. The patient felt that if her husband had really loved her he would have lived to make the trip. His delaying it until his retirement, and its cancellation by his sudden death was proof to her that he never really loved her.

Consider the obviously handicapped person who finds that he is repeatedly turned away when he applies for admission to schools or for job employment. He may very well attribute his inability to be successful to his personal appearance, even though this may not be entirely true. Young adults who have severe acne, stutter, or are unduly obese have expressed feelings of being shunned and rejected by others. The rejected individual finally makes up his mind (unconsciously, of course) never to expose himself to that possibility again. It is too painful to have to cope with the feeling of rejection. In his mind, it would be better to push others away, prevent experiences—in essence, avoid life—before he suffers more hurts. The patient loses all his confidence in others and cannot believe that anyone really is sincerely interested in him as he is now, or ever could be in the future. Furthermore, he will not give you, the doctor, family, or friends, the chance. Why should he, when people have always failed him before? When you approach him, he says that you are staying with him because it's your job and you're getting paid, or because your superior has told you to do so. Your motives are always questioned. He projects onto you what he really feels about himself. One young woman said, "You don't really care; no one ever has." Another said, "Why bother with me? There are others you could have fun with." Both individuals saw themselves as unlovable, unacceptable, worthless people, not significant enough to be given genuine attention. The worker was therefore seen as uncaring, and perhaps playing with the person's feelings to amuse himself.

It is not uncommon for these patients to be extremely sensitive, to make gross misinterpretations, and to attach personal meaning to everyday occurrences. A patient who was last on the list of those scheduled for electrostimulative therapy interpreted this as meaning that the doctor thought the least of her. One patient resented a lack of individual attention from the doctor following his participation in a course for family physicians. This was interpreted as a slight, because the patient felt that the doctor was pleasant at first only so he could use him as a guinea pig, but now had abandoned him. In another instance, an unanticipated change in the scheduled time for a group meeting precipitated a strong reaction in which one patient accused the nurse of deliberately trying to "get rid of" her. Scheduled vacations of personnel often create crises as the patients feel they are being deserted.

At times, the professional worker becomes annoyed, irritated, frustrated, and plain tired. He may have spent an inordinate amount of time with one patient, been as therapeutic as ever, and yet was totally unappreciated. Increasingly, the patient's behavior and attitude irritate him. He begins to ask himself, "Why bother?" It is much easier and more satisfying to work with someone who appreciates staff efforts, or at least responds a little. So, the next time he goes around the unit, he inadvertently passes the patient's room. He forgets to ask him to come to the group session, does not remind him that the barber is on the unit, and neglects to include him in patient outings. After all, the worker knows ahead of time that the patient's response will be an unequivocal "no," and he doesn't appreciate feeling rejected time and time again, either. His pride in himself is shaken, he begins to doubt his professional skills, and his self-confidence decreases. If the worker could magnify his own experience a hundred times, he might have some concept of how desperately the patient fears rejection. He must understand that the patient is not rejecting him personally, but is very fearful of any experience or interaction that may lead to an arousal of his feeling of being unwanted. He must remember that the patient has not developed the ability to sustain normal give-and-take in everyday relationships. Like a child, when he cannot have what he wants when he wants it, he feels that others disapprove of him, cannot love him, and are trying to hurt and reject him.

THE APPROACH TO THE REJECTING PATIENT

Recognize how you feel and behave when the patient rejects you. Accept the patient as he is. Make no attempt to change his behavior by telling him for example, that he is sloppy, or that his hair is too long. Do not demand reasons and explanations for his rejecting behavior. Be nonjudgmental.

Offer a relationship. Tell the patient, "I have come to accompany you on the walk" or "I have come to eat dinner with you." If he questions your motives, reply, "I wouldn't have come in the first place if I really didn't want to."

If the patient will not talk with you, spend at least fifteen minutes just sitting quietly and being with him. Keep the immediate environment low-pressured. Do not push the patient to do more than he can; be content with small gains at first. For example, if a patient refuses to go on a walk with the group, you can suggest that he sit alone with one of the health workers on the patio or in the day room. Do not push him to talk if he is obviously uncomfortable. Tell him, "When you feel more comfortable we will talk together again," and do so. When he can tolerate it, encourage the patient to express his feelings in a verbal manner. At the same time, indicate to him that you accept his expressions of his feelings even though you do not always agree with them. This will make him realize that you are not suggesting that he imitate your behavior.

Don't try to interpret the patient's behavior to him. This may increase his anxiety, and possibly interfere with the start of any therapeutic relationship. The patient needs to feel wanted before he can tolerate any threats. Allow sufficient time for progress, even though it may be slow and uneven. Be consistent in your approach. Several attempts, spaced at intervals throughout the day, will remind the patient that you are really interested and will also inject some doubt into his belief that no one cares.

Cultivate feelings of trust. This can be done by using nonthreatening activities in which the patient can achieve some degree of positive feeling, e.g., exercise class, body movement to music group, walks, ball games, shuffle board, bingo, helping with cleanup. Include the patient in all activities. Even though he is reluctant to participate at first, offer him the opportunity to change his mind. Avoid using empty phrases, e.g., "Your skin really isn't that bad" or "I'm sure everyone really loves you." Instead, offer validation of the patient's feelings with constructive measures he can employ, and/or the opportunity to explore his difficulty. State, "Your skin condition must be distressing. Perhaps with medication, treatment, and less tension it will improve."

Always keep the patient informed of any changes in the schedule, forthcoming events, or procedures. Avoid promising what you cannot deliver.

The Hostile Patient

It is usually easy to recognize the hostile patient. His angry tone of voice and facial expression are apparent to everyone. The worker readily observes that the patient is sarcastic, offers unwarranted criticism in the face of adequate staff performance, condemns his surroundings, is uncooperative no matter how simple the task, and is argumentative with little or no provocation. Obvious overt manifestations of his anger may include throwing magazines or pillows across the room, smashing a glass, or kicking a chair. The patient appears to be easily upset, and anything or everything may become a focus for his faultfinding. He does not want to be bothered in any way, and may be actually insulting to those who try to approach him. His choice of language may be colorful and/or vulgar. Covert hostility should be suspected when the patient is excessively polite, yet manages to convey his constant dissatisfaction with everyone and everything.

When confronted with his behavior, the hostile patient may act as if he does not know what on earth you are talking about. Some patients will offer elaborate explanations for their reactions in order to justify them. These supposedly acceptable reasons for behavior that the patient gives himself are called rationalizations. Sometimes a patient will tell the nurse about problems that are unrelated to what really bothers him. This is because the subject is too painful to deal with at the moment. The patient may be unaware or only partially aware of what is upsetting him. Again, if this glimpse of insight is painful, the patient may deny his anger vehemently and refuse to talk at all. Instead, he displaces his anger onto other people (nurse, aide, social worker, doctor), or whoever is working with him and trying to help. Denial and displacement are often observed when a patient suffers a loss (real or imagined) and feels unloved, rejected, and uncared for.

The hostile patient arouses fear and anxiety in the staff on the unit, particularly if he is assaultive. One practical reason why the staff keeps away from the hostile patient is that his behavior and responses are unpredictable. Fear of being physically hurt leads the worker to avoid the particularly angry patient.

Sometimes there is no forewarning that a patient is becoming angry and unable to control his actions. Several aspects of the patient's behavior, however, may indicate the possibility of approaching trouble; for example, a rising pitch of the voice and cutting comments—"You think you know it all"; "Well, if it isn't the big wheel herself." The patient may also angrily refuse to accept medication or treatment, show clenched fists or slap one clenched fist into an open hand as if in a baseball glove. Often he will complain about the unit setup, kick the bases of the furniture, forcefully dump utensils into the waste basket, or just throw things onto the floor. He may walk in and out of rooms, or up and down the hall in brisk fashion, his glance darting to and fro, but particularly toward the exit door. He may ask questions such as "Are the windows breakable here?" or make such statements as "I'll get even with him if that's the last thing I do" or "I'd burn the place down if I had a match." He may also say things such as "They think I'm stupid; well we'll see about that" or "If she thinks she's going to run my life, she's dead wrong."

Another excuse for avoiding the angry patient is that most people do not like their services to go unappreciated. Since some health workers tend to interpret a patient's hostility as a personal affront to themselves, they tend to walk away from the rejecting individual because their own feelings get in the way of their dealing effectively with the patient.

Many of us are not in the habit of dealing with our own anger or that of others. We keep angry feelings inside ourselves where they steadily accumulate—sometimes for so long that a depression results. In effect, depression is anger turned inwardly upon oneself. When these feelings are finally allowed to come out, they may be directed against the dog, cat, spouse, a parent, or sibling—"safe" individuals who will not retaliate and with whom we feel secure. Some people express anger only when with a group of people, so that a response is unlikely. One family stated that their daughter (the patient) always waited for family gatherings to express her feelings that "all people are rotten. No one cares about me. Everyone is a piece of garbage." Some people displace their anger onto an authority figure and, because they fear repercussions, they don't usually verbalize or act out their anger directly, but instead "gripe" to a peer. The assassination of a public figure is sometimes blamed on this type of displacement.

Among the many reasons the patient may have for being angry is the disability created by his current affliction or the threat it has brought to his job or economic status. He may be angry because he has received inaccurate information from professionals in the past, and may complain that he is being hospitalized unjustly and against his will. Past relationships or occurrences at home or at work that have disappointed him may have never been resolved. He may feel anger at having to experience this problem which he never asked for in the first place! Those old angry feelings are now displaced onto people in his new situation, which somehow seems similar to the previous situation. Therefore, certain aspects of unresolved conflicts of the past are reactivated.

The patient's hostility impairs his relationship with others. People turn away in a rejecting manner. This serves as further proof to the patient that the world is mean and uncaring, increasing his anger. For some, being the butt of negative reactions is somehow better than the isolation of no reaction at all. Yet it is not uncommon for patients to hide their hostility from the health worker for fear that care will be withdrawn if they express anger or displeasure.

The patient's hostility may be an outgrowth of childish feelings or jealousy, reminiscent of his not wanting to share a parent. This becomes evident as health workers become very involved with administering medications or assisting another person. The patient, unable to tolerate the workers' involvement with others, may act out in a hostile way in order to get attention focused on himself.

Young adults often become hostile as a result of disillusionment brought about by what they regard as unfair treatment by adults who promised otherwise. They also show hostility when they see flaws in the character of a cherished role model or when they face the inequities and social injustices of the world.

THE APPROACH TO THE HOSTILE PATIENT

Keep the tone of your voice low and well controlled. React to what the patient says with an honest, open, concerned attitude. You must convince the patient that you care, and want very much to understand his problem.

Remember not to take the patient's criticism personally. This will help you not to become defensive. Quietly answer the patient's tirade by offering an explanation for your functions or the hospital routines. The idea is to acknowledge that you recognize his anger, but doubt that it has a direct relationship to you. Then stay with the patient for a few minutes, demonstrating ease and control in the situation. This allows the patient to feel increasingly comfortable with you and tells him that you are really sincere in wanting to assist him.

Allow the patient an opportunity to talk with you and express himself, without having his feelings hurt. You can do this by saying, "You seem to feel as though someone has disappointed you"; or "You sound as if you are upset about having to remain in the hospital"; or "You seem to be saying that I have done you an injustice. I can understand that it is difficult for you to be here. I am wondering how you are dealing with the situation?" Remember, allow the patient to save face. Do not use expressions which shame him, or show your annoyance: e.g., "We don't act that way here"; "That's immature"; "No wonder people avoid you, the way you behave." Such statements are not helpful and prevent further positive interaction.

Listen to what the patient has to say. It is essential that you be absolutely honest in your responses. Stick to the reality of the situation. For example, if the patient yells, "You can't get anyone in this damn place to help you. I rang hours ago," reply, "Although it is only ten minutes since you buzzed, I know it seems longer to you. I'm sorry the staff nurse was too busy to come immediately. But now that I am here, perhaps I can help you?"

Avoid excessive smiling and ingratiating remarks. The danger here is that the patient may interpret such behavior as insincere and feel that he is being laughed at.

Let the patient set his own pace. Asking questions too soon, or giving advice at the beginning of the relationship is premature. Instead, be available at definite short intervals to talk with the patient.

Get help immediately if it becomes necessary to disarm or subdue a patient. (Incidentally, if you fear talking with such a patient alone, always have an assistant with you.) A controlling environment often helps the patient to control himself. Inform him that you understand he cannot control his actions at this time; therefore, you are helping him to do so. Don't humiliate him while applying restraints or giving intramuscular injections. Offer the patient the opportunity of cooperating with you for his benefit. State, "You need this injection. I have to give this to you even if you refuse. So it would be better for both of us if you could cooperate with me."

Reassure the patient that you are interested in his situation. If he screams, "I'm going to kill myself," try to discover what plans he has for doing so. This lets him know that you are not afraid to discuss the possibility that he may harm himself. Try to have him tell you what it is that he thinks is making him so angry. This allows you to work with him to find other less drastic ways to relieve his uncomfortable impulses, and thus lessen his need to hurt himself.

Try to channel destructive energy into constructive areas. Exercise (shuffleboard, walks), simple work tasks (sanding furniture, stamping envelopes, ripping up discarded paper), and sports such as punchball, volleyball, and kickball, all give an outlet for such energy and reduce the possibility of its use against oneself or others.

The Paranoid Patient

People who are overly suspicious of what we do, overly distrustful of our intentions, and who question every pill, sheet, towel, or glass of water that is brought into the room are described as being "paranoid." Some degree of paranoia is found in everyone. There are those who function well in most areas, yet exhibit some suspiciousness when they are involved with others either at work or in social situations. However, when paranoid behavior is carried to an extreme, it becomes trying to the staff, and makes working with the patient difficult. The professional will frequently encounter this problem on the psychiatric unit. In other areas of the hospital, the patient's paranoia is usually not the primary reason for his hospitalization. Therefore, paranoid behavior is often unrecognized as such and may be attributed to the patient's physical discomfort, an unpleasant previous experience, or dislike for a particular staff member. The stressful situation of hospitalization, with its many unfamiliar and unknown qualities, may indeed heighten the paranoid characteristics that have always been present in more subtle forms. It is not uncommon to find out that in the past the paranoid patient was known as an overly cautious person.

There is usually some acceptable explanation for the patient's way of seeing or interpreting events. Attempts to find out what is real and what is fabrication often just bog the staff down in a fruitless and frustrating endeavor. What is important is that the patient's emphasis on these upsetting thoughts, and his inability to change their focus, prevent him from

101

accepting treatment, from being helped, or even from functioning in his everyday living.

When approached, the patient is suspicious of what is said and why it is being said. He questions everyone's motives. He appears very tense and often has a suspecting, angry gleam in his eyes. He does not trust his family or friends, and certainly not the hospital staff members, whom he has never seen or met before. He feels that each worker is out to "get" him, and that his treatment is of the worst kind. He suspects that the water has either been tampered with or poisoned; the medication will "burn out his insides," or is being used to control his mind; and that the food has been harmfully prepared. He is suspicious of anything that requires explanation. He may go on to complain that the room is "bugged," that the telephone on the desk conceals a tape recorder, and that there are plenty of spies around, all plotting against him. He feels that evidence is being collected to be used against him and that the nurses' notes and charts are definite proof of this. Often, he relates that other people in his life (mailman, coworker, instructor) are conspiring against him because they are threatened by his special qualities. He insists that anyone who differs from him is wrong, and that only *he* sees things correctly. Frequently the paranoid patient has strong inferiority feelings, and belittles others in an attempt to defend against these feelings.

The paranoid patient feels unloved and unaccepted, and believes that almost everyone has let him down, has been unsupportive, and has rejected him. He assumes that others are jealous of him, and want to see him fall. He is angry at this world with all its injustices; this world which has misused him and has striven to treat him unfairly. In his eyes, everything bad that happens to him is unrelated to his own actions, but is the fault of others. He attributes to others the power of reading his mind, and accuses them of conjuring up devious ways to take over his life. He also believes in magical qualities, voicing great faith in extrasensory perception, mental telepathy, consciousness raising through the use of drugs and seances.

The paranoid patient often distorts what is going on in order to have events fit in with his scheme of things. He is frequently fixated on a particular idea, and cannot accept the truth even when it is proven factually. He is usually argumentative, and may be easily provoked to violence. His anger may be stimulated by a staff member's pleasant smile which was intended to enhance friendship and communication. He interprets the smile as an indication that he is being laughed or sneered at, or that a plan is being contrived to cheat him, or make him appear foolish. He is also extremely sensitive to anything that he may interpret as a slight. Even innocuous actions may be interpreted as slighting, as when his nurse talks to someone other than himself, or when she fails to say hello to him before greeting someone else, or when she interrupts a conversation with him to answer the telephone. Trivialities are not trivial to him; they are usually blown up out of all proportion. His resultant behavior is usually so offensive and disturbing to other patients on the unit that they attempt to avoid all contact with him and, unfortunately, this increases his feelings of personal rejection.

Working with such a patient presents special difficulties even when carrying out regular procedures that most patients accept calmly, agreeably, and as a matter of course. For example, if the patient needs a routine chest x-ray, he may be leary of it or may adamantly refuse it, saying, "I know what it really is used for." A request for a urine specimen may be met with, "You really think you have me fooled, don't you?" Because he believes people are trying to "put him away for good," he will balk at signing routine consent forms for treatment and medication. He will read and reread the form, replying, "I am not signing without my lawyer." If his admission to the hospital is voluntary, the patient will doubt it. If it is not voluntary, he will indicate that the circumstances under which he has been admitted are proof of evil doings. Even the property sheet is suspect, and is scrutinized elaborately before the patient will agree to be responsible for clothing and personal articles kept on the unit.

The paranoid patient is acutely uncomfortable and is trying to cope with many painful feelings and problems which he cannot presently face. He handles this by attributing his hostility to others. He will completely avoid recognizing his own feelings by stating that he feels the opposite. At times, he will be overtly belligerent. His illness prevents him from being able to comprehend the meaning of his behavior.

THE APPROACH TO THE PARANOID PATIENT

Recognize the patient's situation in establishing your approach. Tell the patient, "It sounds as though you feel that you were forced to come here"; or "It must be particularly difficult to feel that you were not properly informed about what to expect here"; or "You seem to be upset about the circumstances which led to your being here."

Recognize the patient's fear that he is not being treated fairly. Say, "This situation must be very difficult for you"; or "I can imagine how upset you must feel." As staff members develop a relationship with the patient, they may suggest that even if the patient finds it impossible to disregard his paranoid ideas he can at least give some thought to the workers' views of his situation. Say, "I accept your belief that your boss is cheating you. Even so, I'm glad you stopped threatening him and writing obscene letters. I believe that eventually you'll accept our perception that your boss has been very honest and aboveboard with you."

Look directly at the patient. He perceives this as a sign of your concern for him. It also implies that you are comfortable in the situation when you return his gaze.

Establish your role as a professional person. Stress that because he has not known you before this, you can understand his hesitancy in trusting you. However, reaffirm that your interest in him is a professional one. Paranoid patients are difficult because of their reluctance to accept treatment and their lack of motivation.

If the patient is severely paranoid, and is considered harmful to himself or others, he may have to be hospitalized against his will. Legal procedures must always be followed carefully in such a situation.

Allow the patient to inspect his new environment. Let him explore the room, closet, bath, drawers, behind drapes, particularly if he feels someone has "bugged," wired, or tampered with anything in any way.

Encourage the patient to talk to you and the physician. Tell him, "By talking, you will be able to be helped, and thus cut down on the time you will have to spend in the hospital."

Do not humor the patient when he makes irrational or outrageous demands. Instead say, "I am interested in your request for the exterminator, but at the present time I see nothing to support your feeling that you are being eaten by a huge bug." This may allow the patient to express his real fears, which may be related to himself and others in his life. If he accuses you of playing tricks on him, or of having special reasons for saying and doing what is part of your job, explore his previous reactions with him. Say, "I wonder if anyone ever played such a trick on you?" Avoid directing jokes or funny remarks to this patient. He interprets them as an attempt to make him look foolish.

Try to enlist the patient's cooperation in his treatment program. Give him adequate and intelligent explanations for all plans, procedures, and therapies. Truthfulness, consistency, reliability, firmness, acceptance, and understanding are imperative in establishing trust.

If you approach the patient with a medication, walk into the room surely, calmly, and firmly. First tell him with conviction, and not as if you are anticipating difficulty, "This medication is to be taken now." If the patient asks about the effects of the pill, you can say, "It will help you to relax." If the medication is likely to cause any uncomfortable aftereffects, tell the patient, "After a while your mouth may become dry." This will help him realize that you are not deceiving him. If the patient refuses the medication, calmly state, "We don't believe in coercion, but sometimes a person needs help to help himself. If you are unable to take this medication by yourself, I will help you take each dose until you can take it alone." Then give the medication without delay, and with adequate assistance from the staff.

Work with the patient on any problems which he acknowledges. He often believes he is not sick at all and that he needs no help. Do not provoke him or argue with him about his false beliefs. Instead, ask him, "What role do you think you possibly play in antagonizing others?" Reaffirm correct ideas even if they are not complimentary to you. If the patient says, "You are a big one, aren't you?" and you are, reply, "Yes, I am very heavy." False illusions and beliefs (delusions) serve a purpose. They explain fears, unfulfilled expectations, and diminished hopes. Let the patient know that his false beliefs interfere with healthy functioning. When the patient tells you a bizarre tale and demands a response, reply, "I accept what you say, but I cannot find any evidence that supports your belief that someone is after you."

Let the patient know you realize that he does not like to have any limitations placed on him. If he is on an open psychiatric unit, point out its minor limitations, but stress as well the wider range of freedom that contrasts with that on the closed unit. Stimulate his motivation by giving him special responsibilities and by allowing him choices in such areas as group or occupational therapy. But also set limits. Do not allow him to harass others or be destructive to his environment; it is in no way helpful to the patient.

Be aware of your reaction to the patient. Always be courteous, relaxed, and honest. A trusting relationship will help the patient see himself more realistically.

Be aware of your own behavior. The patient watches your every move—when you giggle, cover your mouth with your hand, motion to another staff member, or whisper in a secretive manner. Do not respond when he challenges your self-esteem with angry remarks. Be tolerant of any accusations he makes about you. Do not humiliate him with your reply, but introduce reality whenever possible. Supporting the patient's right to have an opinion that differs from yours encourages his sense of identity.

Limit your interpretations of the patient's words or actions. Do not confront him with his pathology; this is too threatening to his self-esteem. Instead, when he continues to deny problems say, "Your staying in the hospital must mean you think the doctor and the hospital can help you in some way."

If the patient disrupts individual or group sessions by engaging in a monologue, allow him to continue awhile. This makes him feel important. Then, in order to facilitate the group process, comment, "What you're saying is interesting, but it would be better if you would talk a little about your problem so that the group could help you."

The patient may ask difficult but real questions at the time of admission or during his hospitalization. "Am I wrong to think that?" or "Is it crazy to feel this way?" or "Isn't it possible that what I say is true, and that my husband is the crazy one?" You can explain, "Feelings do not make one crazy. Everyone has had different kinds of feelings at one time or another"; or "The answer to right and wrong is not so easily determined. What is right for one may be wrong for another, or vice versa in a different time or place. Deciding what is right or wrong is something that you have to discover for yourself. It may take time." Then reassure the patient that he will have the help of the doctors and the staff, who will relate to him with honest concern for his benefit.

Do not react negatively when the patient expresses aggressive or homicidal feelings. The patient is sensitive to rejection, and has feelings of inadequacy and worthlessness. Be prepared for changes in his behavior when he encounters situations that kindle these feelings. However, if you are uncomfortable with the patient, admit it to him. Sometimes this can lead to a discussion of what provokes the patient to frighten others. For example, a male patient stepped on a nurse's foot forcefully and deliberately. She told him that he was on her foot and that this was painful. When he removed his foot, she discussed the meaning of the behavior with him. As he talked, he revealed tremendous hostility towards women and his need to assert himself when around them, but that he feared doing so.

The Obsessive-Compulsive Patient

When a person dwells so tenaciously on an idea or thought that he is unable to think of anything else, he is said to have an *obsession*. For example, a person may concentrate on the unwelcome and upsetting idea that he has cancer. Then, despite all medical evidence to the contrary, and a diagnosis of sound physical health, he continues to be plagued by the same thought. As a result, his ability to focus on such simple everyday functions as eating, drinking, sleeping, or dressing is impaired.

Sometimes the thought may be triggered by a stressful situation that provokes an association with an unconscious guilt. The person's usual defenses are lowered by the stress, and so the repressed thought pushes through to consciousness. An example is furnished by the woman whose father died suddenly after a brief illness. As a child she deeply resented her father's frequent long absences from home which were necessitated by his occupation as a traveling salesman. She interpreted those absences as his rejection of her. His death triggered the remembrance of her earlier deep resentment. The feeling was intense and unacceptable to her conscious mind (ego), and she then became obsessed with the thought that her father had rejected her. She thus avoided the feelings of resentment that she harbored about her father's death by substituting the more acceptable, but still very threatening idea that he had rejected her.

A *compulsion* is the persistent urge to carry out a repetitious action. In other words, the person must continuously perform the action over and over again in order to manage his anxiety. One patient kept washing and rewashing his clothes. Another kept returning to her room to count all her belongings and make sure they were all in a certain place, arranged in a special way. Still another patient took hours dressing in the morning because of a compulsion to wash her hands over and over again. Such ritualistic behavior acts as a form of self-punishment and atonement and thus serves to undo any misdeeds the person thinks he has committed.

Although obsessions and compulsions may occur independently of each other, they commonly are seen together. When a patient has an obsessive-compulsive reaction, he experiences recurrences of a repetitious thought, as well as the need to perform a repetitive action. One obsessive lady came to all group meetings with pencil and paper. She took notes of everything said, and anything that happened. She also made lists of everything and anything that came into her head. She involved herself in compiling trivia in order to avoid discussing anything that pertained to her situation, problem, and feelings.

The obsessive-compulsive patient tries to hide and/or prevent demonstration of his feelings. He fears losing control. He strives for order, structure, and a sense of sureness. The individual usually appears neat and fastidious. He cannot tolerate spontaneity or unscheduled activities. Requests or changes create a problem because they intrude into his orderliness. The worker can expect an angry outburst accompanied by much resistance if he informs the patient of recently ordered tests, introduces a new activity, or brings in an unexpected visitor. A patient may even become upset if the furniture in the day room or bedroom is rearranged.

Unrealistic goals are often set by the obsessive-compulsive patient. Attempting to reach and maintain these goals causes much stress. One woman could not leave her home unless it was absolutely clean, with the beds made, laundry done, even the silver polished daily. As a result, morning appointments caused such a high level of anxiety that she would become immobilized. By the same token, a male patient worked well into the night for weeks repairing the deteriorated brickwork of his home because the mason whom he had hired did not work to the patient's high standards.

Decision-making presents difficulty, even though the choices are simple. One lady related that her ruminations regarding which brand of fruit cup was best buy for the least amount of money made daily food shopping impossible. Her fear of disapproval if she should make a wrong decision extended to selecting articles of clothing, choosing a television program to watch, or deciding upon a time to shower. If by some chance she did make a decision, she was plagued by constant self-doubt afterwards and dwelt on whether her decision had been right.

A patient may cling to an idea, think of it over and over, and actually believe it, although it has no rational basis (delusion). One patient was preoccupied with the idea that she was the Virgin Mary. In this case the idea was a substitution for an act that was provoking tremendous anxiety and guilt—an incestuous relationship with her brother.

Obsessive-compulsive patients may be observed in bizarre behavior. One patient always stared downward while walking carefully so that he could avoid stepping on the joints between floor tiles. Another bent his knee and hopped after every fourth step.

Sometimes fear is attached to the obsessive idea, as in the case of a patient who was sure he could not move his bowels because he might contract a venereal disease while sitting on the toilet seat. This patient did not defecate for days. His problem was thought to be related to his early childhood, when he refused to move his bowels in order to express anger at his parents.

Is all obsessive-compulsive behavior abnormal? Certainly not! We all know individuals who demonstrate some degree of this behavior. It is the degree of the behavior rather than the behavior itself which determines its abnormality. Sometimes it is helpful. For instance, in order to get through school or some long and intensive training, one usually establishes certain habits. The room may have to be quiet, or very well lit, or there may have to be cigarettes available before one is able to buckle down. Take, for example, a nurse whose job requires her to be an expert in operating room technique, or one who must carry out isolation technique on a communicable disease unit, or one whose responsibility involves the preparation and administration of exact medications at different precise times. In each of the above situations, the exactness and repetitiveness of the behavior are helpful in achieving constructive goals.

However, when one's thoughts and behavior interfere with, prevent, or obstruct functioning so that one is immobilized and unable to participate in his ordinary life, hospitalization may become necessary. The difficulties in working with such a patient become apparent quickly. He repeats the same absurd idea or irrational thought over and over. No matter how the worker tries, he is unable to get the patient to respond to simple reasoning. One patient repeated, "I know they are after me, and I can't get out," as he paced up and down the room. The nurse kindly but firmly pointed out that as far as she could see, there was no one in the room but herself and the patient. She then demonstrated that the door was open for the patient to go in and out as he pleased. Nevertheless, he showed little response, and continued his actions. Another patient related that he was pushing a steel ball and that nothing would help until it was out of his way. Here the nurse attempted to exaggerate the patient's obsession with his delusion and stated, "I really feel for you and so I had the ball removed." The patient appeared startled, then laughed and stated, "Ha, no one could do that; it's impossible." The need to maintain the obsession and delusion had far deeper importance than the worker's heroic attempt at intervention. Certainly the patient's need for the obsession was great enough to make him ignore rationality.

Another problem frequently present is the inability to tolerate any kind of change. The patient is determined to carry on in his own way. One evening before a scheduled psychodrama session, a patient became severely upset because the session would interfere with her plan to play monopoly. She became angry, insolent, and argumentative. Realizing that her behavior precluded her attendance at the session, the worker decided to allow the patient to play her game. At that point, the patient's self-doubt and inability to make a decision created a conflict. She stated, "Maybe, I'll go, if you say it's important. No one tells me anything." Her rage, though controlled, was apparent in her blazing eyes and clenched fists. The worker, realizing the difficulty the patient was now in, used tender comfort and insisted it was all right for the patient to continue her plan for the evening. After this encouragement, the patient finally accepted the genuine approach of the nurse and did as she had originally planned.

Often, patients fear retaliation if they do what they themselves decide, yet when they feel they are being obedient their self-anger is increased and they become defiant, and this leads to renewed fear of punishment. In the incident cited above, the worker's reaction was helpful to the patient since it allowed her to have an experience unlike any which she had known previously, while living with her parents. It also interrupted her usual but unhealthy behavior pattern. The worker commented to the patient about her expression of emotion in order to bring into her awareness feelings that she usually denied. After the monopoly game had ended, she chatted informally with the patient to dispel any fear of punishment that she might harbor.

The worker is reminded that the obsessive-compulsive patient is extremely anxious and seeks relief in the repetitive act. The patient is not conscious of the real cause of his anxiety and subsequent behavior. For example, to relieve his anxiety, one patient deliberately masturbated at the community meetings. He was not aware that his activity was actually an unconscious way of defying his parents.

THE APPROACH TO THE
OBSESSIVE-COMPULSIVE PATIENT

Use a quiet manner when with the patient. Keep the environment as calm as possible. The radio, television, or record player should not be played loudly. A noisy nurses' station is disturbing to the patient. A private room with bath and, if possible, one that is close to the nurses' station is ideal for increasing the patient's feelings of security.

Reassure the patient of your interest in him. Let him know that you desire to work with him in an effort to help him during his hospitalization. Maintain this interest by staying with him at several intervals during your time on duty.

Don't be judgmental, or verbalize your disapproval of the patient's behavior. Since you recognize that the patient's obsessive thoughts and compulsive behavior are a way of managing his anxiety, do not interrupt or attempt to change his activity. This will only increase his anxiety. Help the patient to channel his energy into satisfying activities. The use of non-verbal activities are better for reducing anxiety than verbal activities. Group activities involving dance, exercise, yoga, bicycle-riding, playing shuffleboard, jogging in place, or walking out-of-doors are all helpful.

Help maintain the patient's physical condition if necessary. Limits must be strictly and consistently enforced to prevent malnutrition, fatigue, and lack of cleanliness.

Do not pressure the patient. Allow him plenty of time to eat, dress, take his medications, and report for activities. Do not hurry him. Do not ask him, "What shall we do?" or "Do you want to do something now?" because such questions pressure him into decision-making. Do not insist that he maintain a strict schedule. If he could control himself and his activities, he would.

Help the patient develop confidence in his own choices. Encourage the patient to find answers for himself. If the patient says, "It's up to you to talk to me about my problems," the health worker can respond, "What specific problem would you like to work on today?"

Allow the patient to express his rage. Do not be defensive. Make sure you acknowledge any rage that is realistic and justifiable. One patient revealed her fury at having to wait over an hour for the health worker, who had been detained on an emergency. The health worker discussed this with the patient, agreeing that the delay, although unavoidable, was certainly a good reason for the patient's angry reaction.

Do not confront the patient with what he says or does. Instead, encourage him to elaborate and discuss his feelings further. Allow him to repeat himself over and over again because this helps him clarify his feelings. Help him to identify his feelings by saying, "You feel silent"; "You feel upset"; or "You feel angry." Comment on his facial expressions, grimaces, downcast eyes. The patient usually feels more than he reveals.

Make only reasonable demands and always explain them. For example, it is not reasonable to expect a patient to be punctual for all activities, or to participate in a forty-minute session with you, or to adjust to the unit environment in a predetermined amount of time. Patience and understanding sustained over a long period of time are musts. Because of the long-term nature of the illness, staff members must make a concerted effort to support each other and to relieve each other on a consistent basis.

As the patient learns about his feelings and becomes more comfortable with them, he will be able to channel the discomfort they arouse more effectively. Trying to argue him out of his obsessive-compulsive behavior or influence him with logical reasoning is to no avail, since his problem has an emotional basis.

The Manic Patient

Manic behavior is characterized by generalized physical and emotional overactivity and results from a disturbance in mood (affect). The amount of activity the patient presents varies with the degree of his illness. Thus, mania ranges from mild (hypomania), to moderate (acute mania), to severe (delirious mania).

The manic patient appears elated, is constantly active and talkative, and may be quite boisterous. His behavior is not related to what is happening around him. He has little patience for anything and is easily distracted from what he tries to do. His attention can be directed to anything but is just as easily lost. In the space of a few minutes, he covers numerous subjects, and goes from one to the other for no apparent reason. He is constantly involved in some activity, but accomplishes very little. Sometimes he is so talkative that his speech is not entirely clear to the listener. Depending on the degree of his manic behavior, he may or may not be confused. If he is not confused, and his illness is mild, he usually does not believe he is emotionally ill or that he belongs in the hospital. Patients in moderate to severe manic states may yell, become argumentative and unreasonably demanding. They may also become abusive and resort to pushing, shoving or hitting. Logic is usually absent. Often the patient is grandiose, believing that he is a millionaire or a public official with untold power.

The manic patient thrives on love, affection, and attention. Generally speaking, he is likable because of his responsiveness and outgoing qualities. He is amusing and full of fun. He may speak in rhymes and make puns. He talks up and tells jokes and anecdotes. When he talks he rambles on with little connection between thoughts, and there is little validity or rationality to what he is saying. Sometimes he will go to ridiculous lengths to prove a point. He may name-drop, cite events that never took place, and fabricate people and circumstances. It is not unusual to find that the manic patient may be uncertain about the identity of strangers. He may greet visitors or others on the unit as though they are his close friends.

The manic patient is an eager participant in all activities. He is always ready to go, and has a quick remark or witty reply on hand. He is the life of the community meeting, jumping up without any apparent provocation to dance, sing, or give a speech on any subject that comes to his mind. He appears to have few inhibitions. If allowed, he will take over and monopolize every activity. Once the patient gets started, it is very difficult to interrupt his behavior since he is completely unaware of what he is doing and has usually captivated everyone's attention. But, after a while his very behavior turns people off and they seek to avoid him. What at first seemed cute and humorous becomes irritating and threatening when one realizes that the individual really cannot control his actions. Since other patients are, themselves, striving to control their behavior, they may fear that they will lose whatever control they may have achieved. What is more, their confidence in the staff's ability to provide limits and appropriate intervention measures may be seriously undermined. If some staff members harbor secret wishes that they themselves could be just a little less inhibited, they may even go along with the fun—until it becomes impossible for them to handle it.

Mania may be thought of as an attempt to avoid or deny depression. Often an unhappy occurrence is cited by family members as having preceded the manic episode. For example, one patient was upset when the therapeutic community in which she was living informed her that she was to be trained for new responsibilities. The patient exhibited manic behavior two weeks later. The psychiatric interview revealed the patient's feeling that she would be unable to learn the necessary new skills. She totally lacked any confidence in her ability to cope with the new situation.

The worker may become so entertained by the patient's behavior and amusing tales that he forgets why the patient was admitted to the hospital. Usually it was this very behavior that caused chaos at home, at work, and in relationships. There is also a tendency to overlook working with the patient because he appears to be in such "good spirits" and can "do so much so quickly for himself." One may even get caught up in some of the patient's ambitious schemes, which may range from grandiose land deals or stock ventures to promises of large contributions to the hospital.

A forty-two-year-old man was admitted to the psychiatric unit of a hospital with a diagnosis of mania. Before his illness, he was considered a good husband and provider, friendly and outgoing. In the hospital he was very active, flitting from patient to staff member, asking numerous questions, but never waiting for a reply. Out of the side of his mouth he interjected his talks with imitations of Donald Duck or Bugs Bunny. He walked around the unit whistling, joking, hopping, and skipping. He indulged in anything that caught his fancy. He ate all the food in the unit refrigerator, kept long lists of notes, and wrote numerous letters to friends encouraging their cooperation in his wild escapades and plans. At one unit meeting he pounced into the middle of the group and began to sing and dance. He then became erotic, displaying himself and making lewd remarks, upsetting those nearby. He reacted to direction with an angry outburst and stamped out of the room. He then quickly made light of the entire matter and returned to his previous jovial demeanor.

Another manic patient bombarded everyone in the unit with a stream of long words used in a fast, witty manner. No matter what anyone said, he had a reply that directed attention back to himself, even if it meant introducing a subject other than the one under discussion. He constantly reminded others that his major problem was how to spend his recently acquired $30,000 annual raise. He ate triple helpings at mealtime and yet lost weight. He talked incessantly, kept copious notes, walked around with a pencil behind his ear and holding a clipboard, as if he were involved in an important urgent undertaking. He frequently contradicted himself, but attached little importance to this when it was brought to his attention. He informed the staff that the physician was planning special treatments particularly for him. When the staff checked on this they found it to be untrue. At one large group meeting, other patients told him to give someone else a chance to express an opinion, and the patient left the meeting, saying that he had to go to the bathroom. Instead, he proceeded to make several telephone calls. He returned at the end of the meeting, and immediately began to talk about his sexual escapades in an exotic country.

Both of the above patients benefitted from the structured program within the hospital unit. Their overactivity lessened as they regained control.

THE APPROACH TO THE MANIC PATIENT

Try to protect the patient from undesirable effects of his behavior. Be aware that he is easily distracted, and may need assistance in the activities of daily living. He may need supervision to insure an adequate food intake and to help him relax. It is important to reduce such exciting external stimuli as loud sounds, bright lights, flurries of activity.

Staff members must be available to the patient at all times. They should be supportive in a quiet, calm, understanding manner. A consistent approach from the staff is vital so that the patient can begin to formulate realistic expectations concerning reactions to his actions. Spend frequent, short periods of time with the patient even if you feel nothing therapeutic is taking place. Your presence is supporting and demonstrates acceptance of the patient.

Help the patient modify his behavior along lines that are socially acceptable. Be alert for sudden mood swings from exhilaration to anger. When the patient is behaving in a manner that may prove embarrassing to him, isolate him until he is able to control himself. Set reasonable limits for him. As the patient gains ground (becomes healthier) and is able to relate his difficulties, let him know that his joyous mood and joking behavior do not appear to be in keeping with the sad story he is telling.

Be aware of yourself. Do not encourage or react to the patient's risqué remarks, coarse jokes, boisterousness, or pranks because you are having a good time or would like to indulge in similar activity.

Do not take offense, argue, or react negatively when the patient becomes angry, argues, or makes unkind, cutting remarks. Instead, say to him, "You must be feeling uncomfortable. Tell me what happened." Then stay with him and provide a calm atmosphere for talking.

Do not encourage or respond to promiscuous behavior. Effect a therapeutic atmosphere by redirecting the patient, in a firm but kind manner, to socially acceptable activity. Tell the patient, "I will help you put your clothes on. Then you and I will be able to go for a walk on the grounds."

Help the patient to rid himself of pressure when he is in an excited state. Divert his attention with repetitious tasks; for example, tearing foam rubber in occupational therapy, sanding wood, assembling charts.

Keep the patient out of group therapy at the beginning of his treatment. His talkativeness and rapid sequence of ideas is disruptive. He may be hurtful to others by citing their shortcomings and, in so doing, prevent others from looking at their own behavior or problems.

Provide the patient with privacy during interviews. Since he is covering up much unhappiness, do not be surprised if he cries. Provide warmth, understanding, and acceptance.

The Patient
with a Psychiatric Emergency

The health worker will often become involved in an emergency psychiatric situation. Such emergencies occur when an individual (or several individuals) experiences so much anxiety that his thinking, actions, and total organization become seriously affected, and he cannot assume any responsibility for himself. Thus, he arrives at the hospital unit accompanied by friends or relatives. Sometimes the patient arrives at the hospital unaccompanied.

Usually, everyone in the situation is under a great deal of stress and appears very anxious. Often the patient cannot communicate adequately, coherently, or effectively. He is unable to state just what is bothering or troubling him. All that comes across is that he expects you to do something to make everything all right again. He may even cry out, "Just help me." He seems to expect a magic, instant solution which will resolve all his problems without the necessity of his revealing anything. Of course this is not possible. At this point, the health worker must talk with the accompanying friends or relatives to obtain some understanding of what may have happened that led to the patient's present state. At the same time, if the patient cannot control his emotions effectively the health worker may need to provide some effective restraints.

The health worker who interviews the patient and/or accompanying relatives or friends needs to assess and explore the situation without becoming unduly upset himself. In other words, he must be calm. If he becomes anxious himself, he will not be able to perform effectively and competently. It is imperative that he impress others with his command of himself and his control of what is occurring in the immediate situation.

There should be professionals who have been trained to treat patients with psychiatric emergencies available to health personnel working in emergency room settings. In addition, emergency room staff should receive specific help with their own reactions in order to offset their anxiety. Often the workers have to deal with a multitude of emotional problems shown by patients brought in by police, social workers, or friends. It is unfortunate that some health professionals in emergency rooms do not recognize the importance of their roles in saving the life of a psychiatric patient. Their help is as necessary to the emotionally distressed person as it is to the patient with a medical problem.

Psychiatric emergencies require immediate attention. It is important to focus on the behavior of the patient, as well as what caused it. A patient may have been exhibiting destructive behavior without receiving any medical attention. However, as soon as his behavior affects someone else, the family is likely to respond. For example, one man had been abusing medication for a long time, but it was not until he threw a lamp at his mother that the family dragged him to the emergency room for help. On the other hand, a patient in the emergency room may seem very subdued; yet the police may report that just a few moments earlier, he attacked an innocent pedestrian.

Every health worker should be aware of the patient's physiological condition. It is not unusual to find that a brain tumor will reflect itself in a patient's unusual behavior. It goes without saying that every patient should be evaluated by a knowledgeable professional.

Initially, the health worker gives the patient the opportunity to talk and tell about the events that made him feel he needed help. Often the patient will relate that "it was all too much," or that he felt he "couldn't continue like this any longer."

The health worker should inquire how the patient arrived at his present state and whether he thinks the problem is an emotional one. If the answer is affirmative, the patient should be asked what makes him think so. This gets the psychiatric nature of the difficulty out in the open and clears the way for the patient to relate some of his unpleasant thoughts and feelings. Often he declares that he is unable to function because he cries all the time, as did a sixty-year-old man following his retirement. More often he will reveal suicidal thoughts and fear of losing all self-control because he has engaged in impulsive acts in which he threatened, hit, or struck out at himself or others. Many patients will say quite openly, "I can't think straight"; "I just can't get myself together"; "I feel like I'm falling apart"; "I can't remember the simplest things, and I forget what I'm doing when I'm in the midst of it"; or "I know it's in my head because I'm so miserable and don't know why."

If possible, it is most helpful for the health worker to obtain information about some of the occurrences that preceded the illness. It is not uncommon for the person involved in an emergency situation to be in a very depressed state. The depression can be the result of the loss of his mother, father, sibling, or even a pet for whom his attachment was so strong that he feels completely lost now that his loved one is gone. A very dependent person may feel that he can no longer continue living without the support of this most important individual. One such case involved a single girl whose closest girlfriend became engaged and planned to marry soon.

Incidents in which a person loses self-esteem and confidence to the extent that he feels demeaned can also precipitate a severe depressive reaction. Such situations may include not being chosen for a much desired promotion, losing a job, being asked to leave school, or breaking up with one's boyfriend. The patient may relate that he feels totally hopeless and that he is contemplating suicide. Often by the time the health worker on the unit sees him the patient has made a suicide attempt in the hope of ending his severe emotional tensions.

Another type of emergency situation involves the patient who is overwhelmed with anxious feelings that make him unable to control his impulses. For example, a man leaving on a vacation with his wife became fearful that he would strangle her when they were alone together. A mother feared she might do harm to her children. A student found his learning ability impaired and feared he would fail all his courses and be dismissed from the university. A woman was deserted by her husband, and became frantic at the prospect of managing herself and her children alone and of being regarded as a failure. A man became overwhelmed with guilt and anxiety at the prospect of taking care of his ill wife; he felt that he would not be able to cope with the situation.

A current situation may also arouse fears which may not be recognized by the person involved. All he knows is that he has distressful and uncomfortable feelings which may be incapacitating. A somatic reaction may occur, and affect him in such a manner that he is unable to walk, faints or falls, or is unable to use an arm, to swallow, or to speak. It is not unusual to see an upset, bewildered family following the health aide who is wheeling such a patient into the psychiatric unit for admission.

The health worker who admits the emergency patient to the hospital can assume that the patient, whether or not he accepts the idea, realizes he needs help. This is definitely so in a voluntary general hospital. The patient anticipates what will happen, particularly if he has had an un-pleasant prior hospitalization or in any way identifies hospitalization with mistreatment. He looks to the worker as one who will help take care of him and provide relief for his distress. Some of his anticipations are valid, while others are based only on his deep, unconscious needs. The valid expectations can be immediately acted upon by the health worker. But those which are products of unrealistic wishful thinking may be impossible and may never materialize. The worker can reassure the patient about what is realistically available, thereby reducing the patient's anxiety and lessening his depression. Although immediate solutions to problems may not be possible, the health team must stress that while he is in the hospital, the patient will be helped to understand himself. Hopefully, he will eventually become strong enough to make his own decisions and to cope with the reality of difficult and unpleasant situations. Once the patient begins to recover, he is more able to accept limitations imposed by life situations, for he realizes that there are alternate plans available for living successfully and comfortably.

The health worker proceeds to admit the patient as calmly, quickly, and with as much interest as is humanly possible. He extends every effort to make the patient feel at ease, and to convey the impression that he knows what he is doing and is in full command of the situation. If the pa-tient is up to it, a brief history of problems and precipitating circum-stances should be obtained. The patient is given every opportunity to talk about what is on his mind and to discuss his feelings and problems. It is also desirable to take him on a brief tour of the unit and explain hospital policies. Reassurance and information regarding the kind of help the patient will be receiving does much to alleviate his fears and unfounded expectations. Some patients expect to be locked up, tied down, physically abused, and denied visitors, mail, and their own clothing. Knowing about the frequency of visiting hours, the necessity for adequate everyday clothing, and the advantages of the hospital environment in helping to reduce tension does much to calm the patient, to establish rapport, and to gain his trust.

Often the worker will have to anticipate the needs of the disorganized patient. In the emergency situation, the health worker assumes an active, assertive, and directing approach. If the patient physically lashes out or becomes violent, additional help may be needed to restrain him until he becomes manageable. The admission procedure should then be continued and the patient queried about the incident. By showing a willingness to understand, the worker often enables the patient to reveal more of what bothers him. The patient may be able to describe the way in which he sometimes upsets others, as well as difficulties he has in controlling himself.

Sometimes a patient balks at accepting hospitalization. There is a moment of, "I don't want to. Oh, no, I'll manage alone"; "What will everyone say?"; "What does it matter; I'm sure I'll never get well"; "This is the end of the line." The worker's attitude and efforts should be directed to persuading and encouraging the person to accept admission, since it may have been decided on as a last resort. If not admitted at this time, the patient's only hope for care may be destroyed. It may confirm for him that no help is available—that he is totally abandoned.

Psychiatric emergencies are crisis situations. This means the patient is unable to solve his problem by his usual means of coping. Therefore, he feels that the problem is insurmountable. The patient requires immediate intervention in terms of decreasing the environmental stimulation. He needs help in pinpointing what is happening currently in his life. It is important to establish which people are closest to him, and to engage them in the formulation of an immediate plan to provide support and guidance until the acute emotional state subsides.

The health worker may, on occasion, receive telephone calls from patients who present an urgent situation. They may state that they are going to kill themselves or someone else, or that they have taken an overdose of pills. He must give immediate attention to these calls since they, too, may be a person's last resort before either killing himself or completely losing control over his impulse to destroy others. When such a call comes to the hospital unit, the health worker must have a quiet place in which to handle the emergency call without distraction. He must keep calm and obtain the caller's name as well as the address and phone number from which he is calling. It is also advantageous to obtain the name and telephone number of nearby relatives or neighbors.

If the patient states that he has taken an overdose of some drug, obtain information regarding the drug taken, the amount, and the time it was taken. The worker should tell the caller that he is going to have help sent directly to the place of the call and that he will call back immediately after arranging for help. If the person objects to giving information or to having help sent, the worker should tell him that he must want help or he wouldn't have called, and in order to receive help, the person must supply the needed information. The worker should inform the caller that he may have swallowed a lethal dose of pills and that action must be taken immediately to save his life. The worker should stress that he will continue to help and, if the caller still refuses to say where he is, the worker should continue to talk to him while someone else makes arrangements to have the call traced.

A final word about patients who present themselves at the clinic but who are not admitted to the hospital unit. Make sure that a plan is formulated before the patient leaves, initiating help for him. Relatives and friends who accompanied the patient to the hospital should be involved. The plan might entail arranging transportation to and from the clinic so that the patient can keep future appointments, or providing for child care, or for someone to be at home with the patient on a temporary basis. Arrangements for a leave of absence from a job or school may also have to be made. Realizing that help is really available encourages the patient to keep his next appointment. However, in spite of such efforts, there are some emergency patients who subsequently change their minds and refuse any help which is offered. These patients should be advised of all resources available to them should they desire help in the future.

THE APPROACH TO THE PATIENT
WITH A PSYCHIATRIC EMERGENCY

Maintain a calm, collected, and assured demeanor. Show sincere interest in the patient and his problem. Do not allow yourself to be upset by the emergency. Encourage the patient to accept hospitalization and offer reassurances by telling the patient, "You will feel better in the hospital, and will be able to resist your impulses, eliminate the voices you are hearing and the unpleasant thoughts you have." Also tell him, "You *can* be treated, and will recover as many other people have."

Sustain the patient in his need to be dependent. Offer him any necessary assistance. If he is crying, offer him a tissue. If he is hungry or thirsty, offer him food or drink. If he is unable to stand securely, offer him an arm to lean on. If necessary, help him remove his outer clothing. If he is unable to reach a decision, or make a selection, take over for him.

Talk with those who accompany the patient, and include them as resource persons. They are often invaluable in helping to formulate a follow-up plan.

Allow privacy so that the patient can speak to you alone. But do not add to patient's fears by blocking or closing the door to the room in which you are talking. This can make the patient feel trapped, and can provoke violence.

Be direct in your approach and assess the potential for suicide. Ask the patient, "Have you ever attempted suicide before?" "Do you have thoughts of suicide now?" Be alert to a family history of suicide or actions of the patient which indicate that he expects not to live—for example, planning to sell his house, giving away jewelry, writing letters to deceased persons, and taking out an insurance policy.

Reduce the patient's anxiety by discussing some of his symptoms. Telling the patient to "try and take it easy" is totally ineffectual. But telling him, "Sometimes if a person is upset he may have a rapid heartbeat, breathe more quickly, or feel faint," helps him to understand what is happening. If he is very confused, introduce yourself by name and role each time you approach him. Attempt to eliminate distractions and get the patient to look directly at you as you talk to him about what is happening.

Reduce the patient's fears by pointing out the reality of what is happening. Or elicit from him what he thinks will happen and what he anticipates it will be like. For instance, if the patient fears that he will lose his mind, the worker can point out that his fear is due to his discomfort, and that preventing and arresting further discomfort will lessen and perhaps eliminate the fear. The patient may also feel that he can never leave the hospital if he accepts admission. Reassure him that he can leave a voluntary unit under his own signature, if accompanied by a relative or friend.

If it becomes necessary, obtain an order for medication with which to calm the patient.

The Patient Receiving
Electrostimulative Treatment

Physicians administer electrostimulative treatment for several psychiatric illnesses. The health worker must be able to respond intelligently and knowledgeably to the patient's questions and concerns about the treatment. He must also be able to reassure and care for the patient adequately. In addition, he should be able to convey what he knows to the patient in easily understood language.

Electrostimulative treatment (EST) has previously been called electroconvulsive treatment, or electric shock treatment. The former names cause many people to remember past accounts of psychiatric patients being dragged off to the shock room against their will, forcibly restrained, and then punished for their behavior. Barbaric, inhumane scenes were depicted, with uncouth attendants showing disdain for the patient's well-being. It is not surprising that such portrayals persuaded many already frightened people not to accept treatment. Even in this day of enlightened medicine and psychiatry, when the doctor tells the patient that he recommends electrostimulative treatment, the patient and his family may react with surprise and horror. They cannot believe that what they consider to be a barbaric measure has not been replaced by something more humane. They may question the wisdom of the treatment and strenuously object to it.

Even without this inference of medical incompetence, the patient has enough problems in handling his anxiety and fears. The dread of becoming unconscious, of being electrocuted, of sustaining brain damage, or of totally losing both mind and memory are now added. The patient has either seen or heard many tales of people who underwent such treatment. He may have watched television or horror movies which conveyed misinformation and half-truths in order to enhance the drama. More recently he may have read that EST has been used on political prisoners to modify their thinking. No wonder he is scared to death.

In order to be of any help to the patient, the health worker needs to be knowledgeable about the treatment and about how to approach the patient to give him emotional support before, during, and after the treatment. Because the trend is for general hospitals to include a psychiatric unit, it is not unusual for a patient in the general medical-surgical area of the hospital to receive treatment. In these selected cases, the patient is brought to the psychiatric unit for the treatment and then returned to his original unit. The care of these patients is the responsibility of the staff on the floor to which the patient is assigned. For this reason, understanding the care of the patient receiving electrostimulative treatment is important not only to the psychiatric health worker, but to all other health workers as well.

Electrostimulative therapy is the conduction of an electric current through the head and brain, using electrodes applied by hand to the temporal portions of the scalp. An electrolytic jelly or paste is used to facilitate the conduction of the current. The range of volt settings varies from 100 volts to 150 volts for 0.75 seconds to 1.25 seconds. The actual voltage, and the time interval used, is determined by the physician. The treatment has been used for acute and chronic endogenous depression, catatonia, involutional melancholia, depression occurring in psychoses such as manic depressive illness, acute schizophrenic episodes, and illnesses unresponsive to medication or psychotherapy.

Many theories have been proposed to explain the reason for the effects of the treatment. No *one* theory has been accepted as the last word on the subject. The more generally accepted explanation is that the current causes a massive discharge of brain cell activity, thereby interrupting established nerve network connections. It is hoped that this will free the patient of some previously painful and undesirable thought and behavior patterns and allow him to form more helpful and desirable connections and patterns. There is no medical evidence that electrostimulative therapy damages the nervous system. Medication is given before the treatment to reduce convulsive muscular movements of the body to mere flickers of movement. This virtually eliminates the danger of fractures.

As a result of the treatment, depression should subside, anxiety should be reduced, and disturbing or recurrent thoughts that have bothered the patient should be interrupted. The number of treatments varies with the individual patient, but generally a series of four to seven are ordered to be administered on alternate days, three times a week, until the series has been completed.

The patient who agrees to a course of electrostimulative treatments can be expected to harbor numerous fears and apprehensions before and even during the series. Some of these fears and apprehensions are also partly related to the emotional illness itself. But those related to the treatment can be worked through with the help of the informed health worker, who can instill a sense of positiveness and hopefulness. Optimism based on new goals, improvement, and eradication of distressing symptoms can be conveyed. In order to get this feeling across to the patient, the worker must first work through his own feelings regarding electrostimulative treatment. For instance, a fearful nurse, or one who thinks of the treatment as awful, or one who blames this treatment for a patient's continued illness, will not be able to be genuinely supportive. Each health worker should avail himself of the opportunity to observe electrostimulative treatment. This will help him clear up his own misconceptions. The rapidity of treatment and the often mild reaction of the patient usually comes as a complete surprise.

The health worker does not aim to alleviate all anxiety before treatment, because that is an impossible and unreachable goal. Rather, he appreciates the patient's feeling of anxiety before treatment as a realistic one that is due to lack of familiarity with the procedure. At the same time, he lets the patient know that it will be possible to cope with this anxiety as he learns about what will happen. The worker can also elaborate on the beneficial effects, and reassure the patient that his anxiety about the treatment will diminish with time.

A major apprehension and concern is that of being put to sleep and being unconscious, with no control over oneself. The patient's concern can be eased somewhat by explaining the controls employed on his behalf until he awakens. His security can be increased by pointing out the presence and the functions of the psychiatrist and other personnel in the treatment room.

On the other hand, some patients who fearfully recall treatment they received years ago, before the use of anesthesia, are totally relieved when they learn that all they will feel is the sensation of having a needle inserted into a vein (such as in a routine blood test), and that they will promptly fall asleep. The health worker has a moral obligation to prepare the patient both physically and emotionally for treatment. The physical preparation is not unusual, with the patient remaining in comfortable, casual clothing. The worker should assume a matter-of-fact but concerned attitude towards the patient during the preparation.

Because of the use of anesthesia, the patient should have nothing to eat or drink after the midnight before the treatment, which is usually given in the early morning. The health worker should be alert to the possibility of patients hiding snacks in their rooms, borrowing food from the other patients, or gulping water while brushing their teeth. Remind the patient to empty his bladder, since the muscle relaxants given can cause incontinence if the bladder is full. Contact lenses must be removed. Eyeglasses are left in the patient's room or removed at treatment time. Women should not have curlers in their hair. A patient who is extremely upset may be given an intramuscular sedative half an hour before the treatment.

The patient is put to sleep before the actual treatment by an anesthesiologist using an intravenous injection of a short-acting anesthetic such as Brevital (sodium methohexital) or Sodium Pentothal. This is followed by a muscle relaxant, Anectine (succinylcholine chloride). Because of the combined use of an anesthetic and a muscle relaxant, body movements are appreciably diminished and major convulsions are rarely seen. The patient's respiratory rate, blood pressure, and cardiac status are monitored throughout the treatment to make certain that he is not in any danger. His brain waves are also monitored to ascertain that a seizure has been induced. Only a stiffening of the body, and a flexing of the feet inward and downward, is visible. Ventilation of the patient is done mechanically until the muscle relaxant wears off and the patient begins to breathe on his own. He awakens in several minutes, and appears groggy and dazed. On returning to his unit from the treatment room, the patient usually sleeps for an hour or so. Frequently, patients are fairly alert and react quickly, needing little rest.

Common physical complaints following treatment are nausea, headache, and muscle stiffness. The health worker should listen carefully to the patient and evaluate each complaint seriously. He should never assume that the patient's complaints are due to the confusion which may follow the treatment, since this attitude not only undermines the patient's confidence but encourages other staff members to doubt the patient's credibility. Many a health worker has, in addition, discovered a more serious problem than that of the initial complaint.

One patient complained of nausea, general weakness, and pain across the chest which bothered him when he breathed. The alert health worker took the patient's vital signs, put him in an upright position, and called the medical doctor. He came immediately, and confirmed the diagnosis of heart attack. However, when complaints are of a minor nature, the patient can usually be reassured that the discomfort is not unusual and medication is available to remedy the temporary distress— aspirin for headache, Compazine for nausea. He can be given a warm bath to relieve muscle stiffness.

On awakening, patients may not recall where they are or why they are in the hospital. Most express concern about losing their memory, and the confusion and strangeness that they feel. They may express surprise that they have already had the treatment, since they usually do not remember receiving it, or even going to the treatment room. Some do not remember events preceding the treatment. Others remember only that a needle was inserted into their arm. Following treatment, patients are prone to forget much about their stay in the hospital, and familiar objects seem strange to them. When out of the hospital on a day's pass, even their homes may seem odd or unusual. Things the patient knew before his hospitalization may be forgotten, as names, addresses, one's age. Some patients do not remember having made telephone calls, whether they have eaten, or conversations with their physician. This lack of mental clarity, and feelings of vagueness and uncertainty may last for minutes, several hours, or days. Although memory impairment is distressing, it is usually temporary. One cannot predict in advance what a patient will forget or remember. The patient should be told that his memory *will* return, and the confusion will clear. In the meantime, the health worker's physical presence and ability to reorient the patient in whatever way he can will help him immensely. The worker's approach to the patient when he wakens should include information on where the patient is, what has happened, and what is now occurring.

The health worker should bear in mind that often patients dwell on their memory impairment following treatment, when in fact the symptoms of their illness have included difficulty in remembering, as well as confusion. Older patients who complain may not recall that they suffered increasing memory loss with the aging process, particularly if they were also depressed. Thus, while the patient's subjective opinion is not discounted, he may have to be reminded that some of his complaints may not stem from the treatment itself. The treatment will alleviate his anxiety and depression, increase his clarity and his ability to concentrate and think, and give him a feeling of well-being.

In the past, health workers have looked upon the patient receiving electrostimulative treatment as nonamenable to other therapeutic activity. As soon as electrostimulative therapy was found to be indicated, the patient was viewed as inaccessible to interaction. He was therefore left alone, which only increased his confusion and state of unhappiness. In a sense, he was isolated and as a result his difficulties increased. We know now that he benefits from an active therapeutic approach. When the patient is encouraged to talk about his treatment, he can express his worries, anxieties, and fears. Answering his questions provides clarification, and sharing his concerns helps him to undergo this difficult experience more comfortably.

If the patient does not remember the precipitating conflict after electrostimulative therapy, or tells you how good he feels and that he is ready to go home, it is best not to remind him of what he could not resolve or what troubled him. Let him receive the full benefit from his treatment, after which he will be better able to cope with gradually returning memories of upsetting experiences.

Inclusion in daily activities, occupational therapy, and group therapy decreases the patient's feelings of isolation and rejection, and serves to increase his reality testing. Having the opportunity to talk about his experiences, sharing his feelings and concerns, allows him to also receive support, compassion, and understanding from others who have undergone, or are presently undergoing, the same therapy. Hearing about something from a person who has had direct experience with the procedure and who feels its benefits is of unquestionable value to a patient.

Families of patients undergoing electrostimulative treatment need enlightened knowledge, intelligent answers, and emotional support to help alleviate their own fears for the patient and to cope with their relatives' reactions. In one meeting held for families of newly admitted patients, family members revealed their feelings of fear and guilt. They felt responsible for subjecting their loved ones to this treatment which, hopefully, would provide improvement, although that could not be guaranteed. Suddenly, one person, a well-groomed and seemingly learned gentleman, revealed that he had received a course of treatment during an acute illness years earlier and had been vastly helped. This revelation so reassured the group that the leaders didn't have to utter another word.

Patients and families often ask whether there is a maximum safe number of treatments and whether a patient can have additional or maintenance treatments beyond that number. The answer is that there is *no* maximum number of treatments. The patient receives as many as are needed to produce the desired optimal effect for him. Some patients may need maintenance treatments after a series has been completed, and they should be assured that these are available. The patient should also be advised not to work, and to allow only a minimum of demands to be made on him during the treatment period. This is especially important if the patient is receiving treatment on an outpatient basis rather than in the controlled environment of the hospital unit.

It is also important to inform both the patient and his family members that although the treatment will relieve his symptoms, it is not a cure-all, nor does it solve all problems and conflicts. However, once the patient is relieved of his immobilizing symptoms, he can begin to work on his difficulties in a more realistic, flexible, and improved manner. To help the patient do this, psychotherapy is strongly encouraged.

THE APPROACH TO THE PATIENT RECEIVING ELECTROSTIMULATIVE THERAPY

Allow time for the patient to discuss and air his feelings before the treatment. Provide clarification when necessary, and correct misconceptions by offering an intelligent explanation of the purpose, the way the treatment is carried out, and the expected results. If possible, an advance visit to the treatment room should be arranged. This often alleviates a distorted mental image of what to anticipate and also gives the patient a sense of familiarity on the treatment day.

Reassure the patient that anyone who is in reasonably good physical health can tolerate the treatment. Tell him that a general physical examination, including blood work, urinalysis, and an electrocardiogram will be done before hand. If anything is found that contraindicates the use of the treatment, the therapy will be withheld. Let the patient know that sometimes physical symptoms result from emotional illness and can be alleviated by electrostimulative treatment.

Remain with the patient before, during, and after the treatment. The physical presence of the health worker is reassuring and necessary on the morning of the treatment. Provide a calm atmosphere; soothing music is allowable. The worker should be familiar with the routine required before the treatment. Tell the patient, "I will be with you during the treatment and will help you until you feel secure and comfortable on your own." Assure the patient that a "hot breakfast will be reserved for after your treatment." This carries the implication that the patient is expected to recover fairly rapidly and will be able to have breakfast with the others in the day room.

Allow the patient to sleep until he awakens after the treatment. On his awakening, reintroduce yourself, with your name and role. Then, reorient the patient slowly to where he is, what he is there for, and what he is to do next. For instance, "You are here at the hospital, and you have had a treatment for your depression. You tolerated your treatment well. I will go with you now to the day room, where you may eat a breakfast that has been reserved for you."

Listen to the patient's complaints, and alleviate any uncomfortable effects of the treatment. Give him medication for nausea, headache, or muscle soreness. Advise him that a warm bath or shower is helpful. Give clear directions and repeat when necessary; the confusion from the treatment may prevent the patient from hearing or understanding your directions or explanations. Help him avoid being embarrassed by this. Understand that he will try to mask his confusion by remaining quiet. Initiate conversation with him, but do not probe or put pressure on him to recall details or past events. Assure him that he will recover his memory loss. Explain his inability to recall coming to the hospital or the events leading to his hospitalization as a desired effect of the treatment. He should not be reminded that he exhibited bizarre behavior or expressed irrational thoughts at the time of his admission.

Protect the patient from making telephone calls or seeing visitors until he has regained control of himself. This may take several hours.

Do not become defensive or argue with the patient when he blames the treatment for all his difficulties and his inability to accomplish anything. Gently but firmly tell him that the difficulties he had before the treatment created unpleasant and uncomfortable symptoms which necessitated treatment. When he uses the treatment as an excuse for his inability to learn, understand, or pursue goals, he can be told, "You will be able to learn more when you have less anxiety. You will then be able to do more with greater ease." Then use a specific example of improvement: "Before the treatment you weren't interested in doing anything. Now you seem eager to finish the pin you are making in occupational therapy."

Stimulate the patient to think about the benefit of some therapy for himself after the treatment. He may say, "Why should I see the doctor? I'm better now." The worker's best approach in this case is to say, "The more one understands about oneself, the better one can handle his feelings and deal with problems as they arise. This means a more enjoyable daily life. You are surely entitled to that."

Include the patient in all activities. Encourage him to do whatever he is able to do—dancing, walking, or engaging in occupational and recreational therapy. Light activity is preferable on the afternoon of the treatment day; the patient will need extra rest. On alternate days, the patient should join group therapy sessions that stress reorientation and the sharing of feelings and concerns. These meetings will diminish his sense of aloneness and restore confidence in his ability to be with others. This generates a sense of function which the patient previously felt incapable of reaching. It also serves to remind him that others are coping with this experience and have been sustained in it. It will reassure him to know that he is supported in his struggle.

The Drug or Alcohol
Dependent Patient

Whenever one uses an unprescribed drug or alcohol on an excessive and continuous basis, one flirts with the possibility of becoming habituated or addicted. One who is addicted, or has a drug habit, cannot function properly or get through his usual day without the substance he craves, and his need for the drug interferes with many aspects of his life. For instance, he may be so physically ill without the drug that he is unable to work. Or, if he is working, he may crave more of the drug to keep up his mood. He may become irritable, nasty, short-tempered, and rude to his friends and coworkers when unable to have it. At home, his family may feel that he is a bit secretive about himself. They don't appreciate his not coming to family gatherings, hardly ever showing up for dinner, and not pitching in with the household duties. But they excuse him because, "Well, that's his nature," and besides he probably is just "going through a stage." It certainly seems that way when one minute he seems happy and content and only a few hours later is miserable and desperate. Other changes may be noticed: his appearance is unkempt, schoolwork suffers, interests and hobbies aren't sustained.

All too often the health worker views the addicted person as resistant, hostile, and ungrateful. This has validity because when a person is under the influence of a chemical substance, he can indeed be difficult, and can be expected to deny his problem totally. This is part of the illness, and demands frequent confrontation by health professionals.

If health professionals are very sympathetic, viewing the addicted person as one who "drinks only as much as I do," or as someone who is "only enjoying himself like my old grandfather did," they are unlikely to convince the patient that he needs treatment and rehabilitation. If, on the other hand, health professionals are judgmental, viewing the addicted person as weak, sinful, degraded, and worthless, they are also likely to be unsuccessful in approaching the patient therapeutically.

Each health professional should develop an awareness of his own attitudes towards drug use. These usually stem from his association with members of his family or significant others whom he may have met through social, educational, religious, political, or professional affiliations. For example, if the health professional had an assaultive parent who abused alcohol, the worker is apt to view the alcoholic as a disgusting, hateful, and fearful person. In one such instance, a staff member became so angry when a female patient arrived inebriated for a group therapy session that he was unable to confront the patient about the way in which her behavior sabotaged not only her own therapy but that of the other participants. By the same token, a worker whose spouse had recovered through a general treatment program that included membership in Alcoholics Anonymous (AA), while she herself had received help in Alanon, was able to be optimistic, enlightening, and helpful to alcoholic patients.

Our society imparts conflicting messages. Drugs and alcohol are all right, but only if you don't get "hooked." Once addicted, the patient is often regarded as hopeless. It is vital that the health worker accept addiction, both on emotional and intellectual levels, as a treatable disease.

The addicted person loses his willpower as a result of the drug or alcohol that he is taking. Most want to get well, but don't know how. The help and guidance of the health worker who has already worked through personal conflicts and received proper education regarding addiction is important. No group, race, religion, or profession is immune to the disease. Everyone is vulnerable. If drug or alcohol use leads to misuse and then abuse, it becomes an illness which can shorten the patient's life.

Some drugs have a calming effect (downs), and others have a stimulating effect (ups). Taking drugs seems to be more common with the adolescent and young adult, while excessive alcohol consumption seems to be more common as one approaches middle age. However, no age group is immune from the possibility of becoming addicted to either drugs or alcohol. It is rare to find a family that has not been personally touched by some aspect of the addiction problem.

What addicts seem to have in common is that they have had some psychological problems before starting to take drugs. Many tried drugs or alcohol to help them cope with their troubles. Some resorted to this in order to ingratiate themselves with their friends. Still others felt that they needed a little lift to help ease some of the daily tensions and ever-increasing responsibilities.

Sometimes the effect of a drug on an addicted individual is visible to others who note a definite change in the person's behavior. The drinker may become very jolly, sociable, outgoing, and assertive. Or he may become nostalgic, sad, weepy, and retreat from others. Users of the so-called psychedelic drugs (amphetamines, LSD, marijuana) hope to feel a stimulating, exhilarating (high) effect. At times, they may have an unexpected effect (a "bad trip"), with terrifying feelings and depression, which may lead to a psychosis.

The benefits of using the drug, says the addict, are the gaining of an ecstatic feeling, a sense of being in touch with one's unconscious, an ability to think better and to relax completely. Whatever a person's reasons for using drugs, there seems to be a relationship between dependency and the personality of the user. The more immature and emotionally unstable the person, the greater the risk of addiction.

Generally, the person who is addicted is one who usually feels "low," centers his thoughts on himself and his needs, is bored easily, has difficulty tolerating any anxiety or coping with any frustrating situations or drives, finds few satisfactions in life, and seeks a continual state of bliss. It is not unusual for the patient to tell the health worker that he was first introduced to drugs by friends and that he really isn't addicted. He will defend the point of view that drugs are helpful to him, not harmful. He will steadfastly maintain that he really doesn't need them, despite the fact that he seeks drugs at every opportunity.

In the general hospital it is not uncommon to meet an addict who was admitted to the hospital for some condition other than his addiction—backache, abdominal cramps, possible gallbladder disease, intestinal obstruction, or a severe headache. Only after nothing is found to be wrong organically does it become apparent that the patient is requesting pain medication every three to four hours.

On the psychiatric unit, the health worker may come into contact with individuals who have developed serious psychiatric complications because of the excessive use of drugs or alcohol. Many of these patients have had long-standing problems due to an unstable personality. The effect of the drug may increase the difficulties, bring out problems that were not obvious previously, or result in a psychosis. One patient, who was experiencing a severe depressive reaction took some drugs, thinking that perhaps they would help her. Instead she had auditory hallucinations which coaxed her to run into the path of a bus.

Whether the patient is on the psychiatric, medical, or surgical unit, the health worker will usually find him very demanding, wanting what he wants when he wants it, particularly his medication. He is easily upset at having to wait, and threatens to sign himself out of the hospital, or calls his doctor, or reports the staff members to the supervisor. His need for attention is always urgent, as are all his requests. He finds the change of shift a particularly desirable time to renew requests and complaints, because the fresh staff is less likely to check thoroughly on how many previous doses of pain medication he has received. The staff may even feel that unless they comply with his demands, there will be a scene which will prolong their time on duty. The patient will tell the staff coming on duty how terrible those on the other shift were. Lying convincingly, he will swear that he has been promised medication anytime he wants it. His idea is to manipulate the staff into meeting his needs through flattery, inducing guilt, or questioning their competence. Incidentally, these patients have a glib tongue and are rather persuasive. Everything they say or swear to should be taken with a large grain of salt.

At the same time, the patient is easily provoked. He will walk away, become angry, yell, become highly indignant and even abusive when he is confronted or thwarted.

Because most addicts deny that they need drugs or alcohol, it is not uncommon for them to resent any help. They often view the health worker as a threatening person, an authority who is out to catch them. Thus the addict may be very careful and guarded with the worker. He does not want to be judged or rejected, as he may have been by others.

The health worker should bear in mind that the addict has developed a physical dependence on the drug. Whether his continued need for drugs results from his psychological difficulties and/or is due to a neurochemical imbalance, which continues even after detoxification, is currently being investigated. If it is due to an imbalance, then the addict will need continuous treatment, much as a diabetic requires insulin. However, regardless of the cause, the health worker's feelings, attitudes, and interest in this illness is crucial to maintaining a sustained and helpful approach to the patient who is addicted.

THE APPROACH TO THE ADDICTED PATIENT

Remember that the patient has a deep problem which he is trying to solve through drink or drugs. Do not moralize or scold him for his behavior. Everyone else has done this, and it does not help. Help him realize that his behavior is a symptom of his illness. He is also likely to be depressed and anxious and to suffer from insomnia, gastritis, and unexplained bruises that are often due to unremembered falls.

Do not directly confront the patient since he has a low tolerance for frustration. He probably will balk and reject any confrontation. This is because the drugs alter perception, making it difficult, if not impossible, for the patient to recall what has happened, especially if he has had a blackout or hallucination. Do not involve him in anxiety-producing situations. Instead, begin with an individual interaction to let him know that you are concerned and interested in him. Discuss his acting-out behavior as it occurs. Help him develop some awareness of his strengths and abilities. This builds ego strength and improves his self-concept.

Remember that treatment is usually long-term and slow. Those who care for the addictive patient must have a great deal of patience. Be aware of your own feelings toward the patient. If you dislike, feel angry towards, or look down on the addicted patient, then do not work with him. Do not argue with the patient when he defends his right to use drugs or praises their beneficial effects.

Realize that relapses can occur, as with any illness. Do not expect the addicted patient to always be in control. Remember that loss of control and an irrational need to use drugs or alcohol is a prime manifestation of his illness.

Set up a flexible but consistent therapeutic schedule. This will provide opportunities for the patient to find ways to fulfill himself without drugs. Promote activities and interests that provide a feeling of satisfaction. Use films and documentaries that do not make drug use appealing.

Educate the patient regarding the disease. Don't advise a patient to "cut down." If he could, he would have done so long ago. This is the crux of the patient's difficulty. Once he starts drinking or taking any drugs, he loses all control and is unable to stop.

Give attention to the patient's physical condition and appearance. Involvement in drug use or alcohol tends to diminish interest in many aspects of self-care.

Remember that most addicts have unresolved emotional problems. Initially, the addict may have used drugs as a way of asserting his independence. He may also have been using them to express anger towards his parents or other authority figures. He may also have deep-rooted feelings of inadequacy, and is using drugs to make himself feel more able to cope. Since drinking or drug use most often begins in the home, family members also need education. Let the family know that covering up the addiction problem out of guilt and shame only adds to the problem.

Firmly but kindly describe any episodes that occurred while the patient was under the influence of drugs or alcohol. If the patient refuses help, saying he can do it himself, encourage him to evaluate his progress at intervals. In time, he may agree to enter treatment.

Be aware of your own drinking and drug habits. Do not use them as a guideline in determining whether or not the patient has an addiction.

Encourage the patient's participation in community groups such as Alcoholics Anonymous. His family should be encouraged to join the companion groups, such as Alanon or Alateen.

The Acutely Suicidal Patient

Although most depressed patients give some thought to suicide, only a few will act on their unhappy feelings. Most will dismiss these thoughts because they fear possible pain when dying, have religious beliefs opposed to taking one's life, or do not want to inflict emotional pain on their loved ones. Others do not kill themselves because they keenly feel their responsibility to children, spouse, or job or other situation. Some are unready to separate from meaningful relationships, while others, even though morbidly depressed, still feel there is hope for the future and help is available.

Some patients, however, always seem to be walking on a thin tightrope, wavering between their unhappy suicidal thoughts and their internal struggle to prevent themselves from acting on them. This type of patient will constantly talk of his wish to be dead, the pain of his meaningless life, his bleak and dismal future, and his rotten luck. He repeatedly states that there is no one and nothing worth living for in his life and that everything he does turns out poorly.

The actively suicidal patient may telephone others frequently to express his thoughts of dying. He may also write long rambling letters in which he threatens to end his life. He may make suicidal gestures, such as using a nail file to scratch his wrists superficially or swallowing an overdose of pills, perhaps asking for more water because they aren't going down right. He may repeatedly bang his head on a wall, or abuse alcohol before driving, to the point where he can become involved in a car accident. Most patients will talk openly about their disturbing thoughts and specific plans for suicide. However, there are those who do not, yet need to be evaluated seriously in order to assess the urgency of the situation. It is important to remember that most patients are ambivalent regarding their actions and usually can be persuaded that they have options other than death.

Suicidal communication is usually a request to be saved rather than a statement of action. However, there are higher suicide rates among those patients with a history of previous attempts or those who have a blood relative who has attempted or committed suicide. Other high-risk patients are those with a close friend who has attempted or committed suicide and those who have lost one or more significant persons in their lives and believe that suicide is a way to join those individuals. Suicide also appeals to patients who believe strongly that death is a pleasant sleep through which they will awaken in a better world and those who feel extremely guilty about past misdeeds and want to end the torture of self-reproach.

Predisposing factors may be traced back to the patient's childhood, when he developed a poor self-image as a result of overcritical parents or the loss of a very important and meaningful person. The feelings which disturbed him in those formative years may be reinforced by a recent crisis in his life, such as the death of a loved one, divorce, school or work failure, severe illness, leaving home for college or marriage, climacteric, or loss of a body part through surgery. The patient who has poor coping skills in dealing with stress is more likely to attempt suicide. He is, in essence, waving a red flag. It signifies, "Stop. Listen to me. I need help."

Health workers often become intensely anxious when hearing the suicidal patient's dialogue. For them, as for most people, self-destruction is contrary to everything they have learned about the sacredness of human life. In addition, they are often intensely involved in helping people fight life-threatening physical illnesses. They often have difficulty in understanding why a physically healthy individual deliberately attempts to end his life and may become angry, particularly when the patient's care necessitates attention that could be given to others who want to live. How often do health workers say, "He just wants attention, that's all"; "She'll do anything to get her own way"; or "How can she be unhappy with all that she has. It must be an act."

It is important to realize that suicidal patients can be intensely fearful of intimacy with others, yet, at the same time are unable to tolerate the separation or rejection which they often invite by their behavior. When placed in a situation with increasing intimacy or the possibility of separation or rejection exists, the patient may panic to the extent that his loss of self-control becomes apparent. One patient demanded that his father give him a lump sum of five thousand dollars with no questions asked. The father explained that he could not do this, but offered a monthly allotment instead. The patient took this answer as a rejection of himself and attempted suicide by taking an overdose of sleeping pills. Another patient took an overdose the day her boyfriend broached the subject of marriage, fearing the intimacy of the marital situation.

The suicidal patient can also be viewed as a chronically depressed person who leans heavily on others and is unable to manage by himself. When alone, the patient appears to break down as his innermost hidden feelings break through to consciousness. An example is the student who was regarded as bright, obedient, and responsible. However, once away at college and separated from her family, who supplied continuous unconditional love, she became severely suicidal.

Hospital personnel react with remorse, guilt, and anger to suicides which occur on any hospital unit, particularly so if they take place in the psychiatric area. In one case, the patient hung himself. The staff members expressed their distress at not having paid more attention to the patient and spent many hours reflecting on what could have been done during the patient's stay to prevent his death. Some staff members tried to lessen the emotional trauma by faulting the patient for his actions. One said, "Too bad he came into the hospital to kill himself. He should have done it at home so we wouldn't have all this trouble."

Health professionals must keep in mind that they are not omnipotent, and many times, despite all their hard work and therapeutic approaches, a patient will succeed in killing himself. At times like this, health professionals must support and help each other to work through their feelings, while at the same time searching for answers which may not be forthcoming. However, open discussion of this failure is important in preventing projection of blame on coworkers, supervisors, the physician, or the patient's significant others.

Suicidal patients *do* talk about their plans. The slightest hint must be taken seriously. Staff indifference or resistance to initiating therapeutic changes are detrimental to the patient's care. Extra staff members should be recruited from an on-call or per diem staff to relieve the regular staff of nonprofessional duties while they direct their energies to managing the patient. Strain and drain on the staff is intense, as the health professionals work closely together in a joint effort on a most complicated problem.

Staff members are frequently fearful that their words or actions may stimulate a suicidal patient to carry out his intentions. They may therefore keep all conversation on a superficial level, avoiding any reference to the patient's problems. Ignoring the problem does not end it. Instead, it further isolates the patient, making him feel even more rejected. He can then review his plans, consolidate them, and collect any supplies needed for his attempt. He may secrete pills in his mouth instead of swallowing them, or hide sharp utensils (knives, scissors, needles) or a rope or belt in his room. A patient at home may decide to clean his guns or take a high-speed automobile drive. It is much better to confront the patient by asking directly, "Are you thinking of suicide?" If the patient says yes, it is important to get further information about his plans. He will probably be willing to discuss what he is contemplating, telling the worker how, when, and where he intends to carry out his actions.

The suicidal patient's feelings of helplessness and hopelessness should be acknowledged, along with the fact that suicide is certainly one option, but far from the only one. The worker can then help him explore the other options that are available. Motivating the patient to mobilize his thoughts in a more positive vein may offer him the first glimmer of help and hope, so that he can move away from his preoccupation with self-destruction.

Not all suicidal behavior is overt. It may be hidden in such subtle ways as to be almost unrecognizable. Some patients appear to be very accident prone, falling down a flight of stairs or in front of a speeding car, later saying that they lost their balance. Others may "forget" to take life-sustaining medications or take double doses. Others indulge in activities which are medically unwise for them. Patients on dietary restrictions may go on a "binge," indulging in substances which are potentially harmful.

The health professional must evaluate the patient's potential for success in attempting suicide. Although women are more frequently involved in suicidal gestures, men are more likely to succeed, as are older or chronically ill patients. Those with specific plans, who have a lethal method available, should be taken very seriously. Patients who verbalize feelings of extreme helplessness, hopelessness, and guilt, particularly in the wake of a significant loss of a meaningful person or life style, are at great risk. In

addition, if the patient lacks a support system of friends, relatives, or professionals, he is even more likely to choose suicide as his only solution.

A patient can be treated on an ambulatory basis if there are involved
people willing to assume responsibility for him in constant attendance and
the patient's main problem does not have a long-standing emotional basis.
More than half of such suicidal patients in the emergency department at
one hospital responded to techniques of immediate crisis intervention, returning for ongoing follow-up care. The therapy was reality based, ex-
ploring the alternatives which were available to the patient.

On the other hand, there are times when immediate hospitalization
is needed to protect the patient from himself or to undo the damage
brought about by self-inflicted actions. This is more frequently the case
when the patient has been emotionally dysfunctional in the past and has
deep-seated problems. The admission may be directly to an intensive care
unit, where the stomach may have to be pumped to remove an overdose of
drugs, or to an operating room to repair slash, stab, or gunshot wounds.
The patient may be familiar to the staff from similar admissions in the
past. If so, they may feel very hostile as he again diverts their time and
energies from others who will appreciate their efforts. It is difficult to feel
a deep commitment to saving someone who not only is ungrateful but
even angry that he is still alive.

On admission a suicidal patient and his possessions must be thoroughly searched for anything which he may use to harm himself. He may
have to give up his belt, razors, mirror, or any other sharp or breakable
possessions. He may have to be observed when undressing and his belongings searched for harmful objects. One woman had hidden a lethal dose of
medications in a vaginal tampon which no one thought to remove upon
admission. She swallowed its contents during the night, nearly dying in the
process. A man had taped a razor blade into the hem of a bathrobe and
slashed his throat during the change of shifts when he knew the nurses
were involved with sharing information. Still another managed to hide
enough rope within a pajama leg to successfully hang himself on the unit's
shower curtain rod. The patient may be very devious in trying to reach
his goal!

Patients may be placed on suicidal precautions in any location—
home, general or psychiatric hospital, or even a jail. The person assigned to
his care must remain alert at all times to a sudden destructive action. One

man who appeared to be improving was left alone while the worker spoke with the physician in the hallway. The patient took this opportunity to dash across the room, hurling himself through a closed window, landing on the ground four floors below. This particular incident should remind health care providers that patients who appear less depressed may be so only because they have formulated a plan for death which they believe will be successful. True improvement is often difficult to assess, but signs should include an increased sense of self-worth, a positive connection with significant others, and a sense that there is hope or options preferable to death. The staff should adopt the view that the patient has a treatable depressive illness and work cooperatively towards his improvement.

THE APPROACH TO THE ACUTELY SUICIDAL PATIENT

Don't become a partner to the patient's actions by promising to keep his thoughts and actions secret. By sharing his plans with you, he is asking for professional intervention, even though he may deny that this is so. Tell the patient, "As a professional, I will never promise to keep such information secret, nor will I ever be a partner to your plans to take your own life."

Take the patient seriously. Ask him if you understand him correctly, repeating what he has said. Do not be judgmental. Rather, let the patient know that you are concerned about him, even though his behavior causes you some anxiety. Remember that inquiring about suicidal thoughts or plans is not the cause of action. The questions are a sign that you are interested and that you have the ability to handle a difficult subject. This will increase his confidence in you. Don't be misled by a negative response, since some patients believe it is useless to discuss their feelings because "nothing can help."

Find out whether people close to the patient are aware of his unhappiness. Help the significant others in his life deal with their feelings about him. Remember, they can be an important support system for him. Check with them as to the presence of lethal weapons or drugs in the home before the patient is discharged.

Let the patient know when you sense he is creating a situation in which he may feel rejected. "It seems that you felt rejected when the doctor was unable to talk with you on the telephone at that moment that you called. Was he rejecting *you,* or being realistic about the lack of time just then? Were you equating his inability to give you immediate attention with your own feelings of low self-worth?"

Rotate patient assignments while working closely with the suicidal individual. This is to help him develop a higher level of self-esteem as several people demonstrate interest in him. At the same time, supervision can be maintained more adequately by staff members who are not lulled into a false sense of security as they become used to the patient's mannerisms.

Be constantly alert to any alteration in the patient's requests, affect, tone of voice, statements or behavior.

Although the patient's environment should be made as safe as possible, keep in mind that restricting him severely may increase his ideas regarding how unacceptable he is and foster impulsive negative behavior.

Approach the patient frequently. Friendly staff will be helpful in assisting him through stressful periods when he feels neglected, as during the nurses' change of shift, nights, or his therapist's day off.

Don't argue with the suicidal patient. This only increases his feelings of being rejected. Instead, stimulate his thinking towards solutions other than suicide.

Encourage the patient to talk about his feelings. Help him identify the precipitating event by asking questions like, "When do you feel this started?"

Convey your belief that the patient will recover and that there is hope. Ask the patient, "What activities appeal to you for work or recreation in the weeks to come?" Remember that although the patient may not be able to think this through or give you an answer, he is not necessarily out of contact with reality. He may just be desperate and overwhelmed by his unhappiness.

Do not tell the patient how improved he is, since he may then feel obliged to make a suicidal gesture to prove that he is still very ill. Allow him to set his own pace and tell you when he is feeling better.

Include the patient in scheduled activities in order to redirect his energy, lessen his sense of rejection, and prevent the isolation that may lead to the formulation of specific lethal plans.

Sleep disturbances frequently cause suicidal patients to awaken early. Be alert to these hours since patients are often most depressed then.

The Patient with Sexual Problems

Knowledge of sexual development and sexual behavior has become increasingly important to health care providers as public standards have changed. Behavior that was once considered perverted is perhaps now regarded only as deviant and may in the future be looked upon as an acceptable alternative to "normal" sexual activity. No longer is sexual behavior an important factor in determining an individual's value, although there is a continuing interest in the acts of private and public figures. In general, people are more willing to accept their own sexuality, recognizing that this is but one facet of their personalities.

Before 1972 scientists believed that an individual's sex was solely determined by the X and Y chromosomes that were linked as the sperm fertilized the ovum. This meant that if an X chromosome from the ovum joined the X from the sperm, a female would result. But if the ovum's X met with the sperm's Y chromosome, a male would result. Although these facts are basically correct, newer information includes factors that affect the intrauterine development of the embryo and fetus. It is now believed that the fetal gonads begin their development as ovaries and that fetal and paranatal androgens must be present as inductor substances to change the fetus to a male. These same fetal androgens appear to help the brain organize for future specific sexual behavior. This provides some clues as to why women receiving certain hormones during pregnancy may deliver children with anomalies of their external genitals. This area is also being explored as a possible physiological basis for homosexual behavior.

Sexual development continues after birth. Infant boys have erections, while infant girls have been observed rubbing their thighs and moving their pelvic areas in multiple thrusts. In both, the activity ends with a relaxed period of sleep. There also seems to be an imprinting of sexual expectations on children from birth by the behavioral patterns of their care providers. Little girls are handled more tenderly, are expected to be more gentle and cleaner, and are frequently dressed in frillier clothing.

From eighteen months to five years, children can be expected to be involved in self-exploration, including their genitals. Parents usually do not voice displeasure when a child feels his nose, ears, or lips, but may pull a child's hands away as he explores his "private parts." This definitely gets a message across—the genitals are dirty, naughty, and should not be touched. The child then meets his first big conflict. Does he provide himself with the pleasure he enjoys through autoeroticism, or should he live according to parental standards? If he chooses pleasure, will he be overwhelmed with guilt?

In today's permissive society, youngsters may become involved in sexual activity as early as eight or ten years of age. Males are capable of experiencing orgasm within two years of puberty, and may engage in masturbation on a frequent basis to achieve sexual release. Girls may become involved in unprotected sex to become part of the "gang," or as a way of attaining closeness.

At present, there are almost a half million pregnancies per year in unwed females, and about half of these are in teen-agers. While some elect to terminate the pregnancy or give the baby up for adoption, most decide, although single, to keep and raise the baby. Often this means the end of the mother's education, sealing her fate in terms of low-level jobs. These mothers have a high potential for child-battering (they, too, were probably battered as children), and are likely to become pregnant again. They may be knowledgeable about the anatomy and physiology of pregnancy, but tend not to integrate the facts that they have learned in sex education classes with the ways in which their own bodies function. Therefore, although they may have learned about contraceptive measures, they do not apply them properly in practice. Many refuse to use contraceptives because they don't wish to acknowledge any thoughts about intercourse. For them, lack of protection is equated with spontaneity of action, for which they do not feel guilty.

Some pregnancies are quite deliberate and are used to prove that the "girl" is truly a woman. For others, having a baby represents an important goal: at long last, the individual has someone of her own to love. Unfortunately, the area of responsibility is not recognized, and little thought is given to aspects of day-to-day care that will be needed by the child. Still others see pregnancy as a hold on a man that will lead to marriage, without realizing that about 50 percent of such marriages end in divorce. Some choose pregnancy as a way to punish overly strict parents, while others may choose pregnancy as a way to meet their own parents' needs to have a baby in the family. (This is particularly true in families where the mother works to provide support and her child is raised by the grandmother. This skipped-generation upbringing deprives the mother of closeness with her own child. In effect, she becomes a sibling to her own child, rather than the parent.)

Coitus used to be delayed until later in adolescence (sixteen to eighteen years), but has steadily been increasing as an activity among younger adolescents. Often the naive youth who is over eighteen finds that he is unprepared to handle the sexual pressures to be found in college life. He may not be ready to become involved sexually, yet may be fearful that classmates will jeer at him for remaining a virgin. As a result, he may develop symptoms that relieve him of the necessity for sexual involvement. He may complain of headaches, gastrointestinal symptoms, or anxiety attacks that allow him to withdraw from social activities. His problems may be severe enough to result in hospitalization, yet so covert that the underlying cause is not suspected.

During the period of more or less permanent relationships, the young adult (twenty-three to thirty years) may enjoy lovemaking or may be so concerned about his level of sexual performance that he is immobilized and cannot perform at all. Both sexes are very aware of their right to orgasms and may complain of feeling inadequate if both partners are unable to reach the common American myth of equal orgasms at the same time. One partner may have a more extensive sexual appetite than the other and may desire more experimentation with different aspects of sexual behavior. This may or may not be acceptable to the other.

Venereal diseases have risen sharply as more individuals are involved with a variety of partners. Gonorrhea is the most common, with an average of ten to fifteen million cases a year being suspected. Of these, 25 percent involve teen-agers. Some organisms which were limited to mouth, anus, or genitals may now be found in other areas, as oral-genital, anal-genital, or genital-genital sex are practiced.

During middlescence (thirties to seventies), sexual performance is often related to work performance. If the individual sees himself as potent in life, he will probably continue to be effective sexually. On the other hand, if he sees himself as having failed, as unable to attain his goals, he is likely to be less able to perform sexually. The longer the period of abstinence, the more difficult it will be to perform well. At this time, male interest may decrease, while female interest increases. The menopause, with its freedom from possible pregnancy, may allow some women to enjoy lovemaking more than ever before. But for others, the end of childbearing, as well as some unpleasant physical symptoms of menopause (vaginal dryness, hot flashes with perspiration, breast and bone pain) may lessen the desire for intercourse.

Sexual activity continues for healthy adults through their sixties, seventies, and even later years. Some are made to feel guilty or ashamed by their children, almost as though they had reentered adolescence. They may lose mates through death or divorce, and choose others. For some, the loss and grief reactions may be so severe and prolonged that restructuring of their lives is delayed for a period of years, or perhaps forever. Again, physical symptoms may be a sign of emotional problems.

In today's society, many sexual variations exist. Sexual identity is determined by the external genitalia—male or female—while gender identity depends on the individual's orientation to the masculine or feminine role. Disturbances in sexual orientation may cause social problems, as the person determines whether he wants to be heterosexual, homosexual, or bisexual. Regardless of his decision, he may be hypo- or hyperactive, or may have problems with impotency. Men may suffer from premature or retarded ejaculation, while females may complain of dyspareunia (pain upon intercourse), vaginismus (contractions of the vagina that may prevent admission of the penis), or orgasmic dysfunction. Some may decide on transsexual changes to reverse what they see as a "mistake" by nature in their sexual identity. This may involve surgery, hormone supplements, electrolysis, and learning the gestures and voice modulation of the chosen identity.

Sex crimes result in severe problems for some patients. Rape is one crime which can involve a victim of either sex and any age. It is unlike other crimes in that the victim is often considered as guilty as the offender, particularly if the individual is a young, attractive, unescorted woman in a locality of questionable safety at a late hour. Health professionals often work closely with law enforcement officials as they question and physically examine the victim. Evidence that can be used against the offender must be saved and handled in a nondestructive manner. Fragments of the offender's clothing, skin, or hair may be present under the victim's fingernails, in her mouth, or vagina. There may or may not be an ejaculate specimen, since offenders are often impotent.

Rape, contrary to common thought, is not a crime of love, but is an act of hostility, meant to hurt and demean the victim. She may be bruised in any area of her body, and may be bleeding from her mouth, vagina, and rectum. Beyond the physical damage, and perhaps more important, is the psychological damage that results from twisting what should be an act of love into an act of hate and pain. The approach of the health care provider should be gentle, understanding, and supportive. The patient should be encouraged to talk about the incident as fully as possible, in order to lessen the possibility of long-term emotional damage. If there has been more than one rapist, each incident should be discussed separately, since the victim's reaction may have differed with each. In one case, the teen-aged victim reacted most hysterically to the offender who initially made her feel that he would help her escape and protect her from further attacks by the others. He then took her to another room and proceeded to rape her. She saw this as more deceitful than the acts of his four companions, who had threatened to kill her as they raped and sodomized her.

Young children present the most difficult problem when they are rape victims, since they may not understand what the brutality meant. They may be the victims of that most specialized form of rape—incest. Again, the victim is usually a girl, and often preadolescent, so that pregnancy is not possible. The emotional load of having a loved and trusted relative take advantage of a child is extremely traumatic. The child has usually been sworn to secrecy, so that telling a parent (or another person) becomes an act of disloyalty. In addition, the child may enjoy the closeness, and be afraid that it will stop once discovered. Another fear is that the offending relative (usually a parent or sibling) may be removed from the home and punished by the authorities. Even if the child does complain, the accusation may not be believed and the child punished for telling a falsehood.

Sexual problems may also result from medical disorders or surgical procedures. Most patients are disinterested in sexual activity when acutely ill, but may be concerned about what the future holds. Many are afraid that health personnel will reject them if they voice worries about sexual limitations. It is therefore important to anticipate such concerns and bring them into the open. Patients with heart disease may mistakenly believe that their sexual activity is ended forever, and may become deeply depressed. Health workers should clarify any prohibitions and make suggestions that will help the patient function in a way that he finds acceptable. Most patients can resume sexual intercourse when they have recovered to the point where they can climb stairs and walk rapidly. Some may require nitroglycerine before sexual relations to prevent angina. Comfort may be increased if the partner is on top and assumes most of the physical exertion.

Other medical problems, such as radical surgery for cancer, may result in castration. The patient and his mate should then be encouraged to explore various ways of finding (and providing) sexual satisfaction. Kissing, touching, and physical closeness may become as meaningful as intercourse. The absence of a penis, testicles, uterus, vagina, or breast will undoubtedly affect the individual's vision of himself. Plastic surgery or prostheses have been used successfully to refashion missing parts, but the resulting emotional state is even more important for most patients. Much help may be needed to help the patient recognize his own continuing worth in light of his changed body. He may need tremendous support to believe that life is still worth living.

Reproduction is another area in which sexual concerns abound. The very state of pregnancy may cause emotional problems for the mother- or father-to-be. Even when a pregnancy is desired and planned, it may cause a high level of anxiety as an acceptable life style is changed. This is particularly true when a woman is involved in a successful and satisfying career. It also occurs when there is a history of previous miscarriages, loss of a fetus or child, previous birth of a child with anomalies, or a period of infertility. The couple may be supportive of each other as they endure limitations of sexual activity or are concerned about what the future holds. Perhaps the greatest difficulty occurs when a fetal death has taken place and the mother is told that she must wait until labor starts in order to deliver a dead baby. She may be asked to wait at home, possibly for several weeks, before delivering. This is considered the safest procedure in terms of the mother's physical state, but is devastating emotionally. Those who are unaware of what is happening will continue to inquire about the pregnancy. Others who do know may avoid her, fearful that any questions will distress her. In either case, her reaction will be an indication of her deep emotional turmoil. The fact that she has a dead body within her uterus is understandably unacceptable. Most women in such a situation are deeply sedated for the delivery, since the fetus will probably be macerated and odorous. They need to talk about the event and their feelings, and should be warned that they may have nightmares about the event, difficulty in sleeping (perhaps to avoid the bad dreams), and marked depression as they work through their feelings of grief. Almost all search for reasons and may not be satisfied when none are available.

In order to help patients with sexual problems, health professionals need to have a positive sense of their own sexuality. It takes practice to be comfortable when discussing such matters, particularly if one has many inhibitions in this area. This does not mean that the professional has to be sexually active in order to help others, any more than one has to have an infarct, a stroke, or cancer before counseling patients with those disorders. The health worker can learn a great deal from reading on the subject, as well as from watching films geared to providing helpful information. The more knowledgeable the worker, the more valuable his input will be.

THE APPROACH TO THE PATIENT
WITH SEXUAL PROBLEMS

Be available to patients who want to discuss sexual problems. There are several national organizations with local branches which can provide additional information and specific help.

Recognize the possibility of sexual problems resulting from medical disorders or surgical procedures. Help the patient verbalize his feelings.

If the patient is a victim of rape or incest, collect and label physical evidence carefully and keep it available for law enforcement officials. Be supportive, encouraging the patient to discuss the situation as fully as possible. Keep a written record of the patient's description of the persons involved or of the event, since the patient may be unable to recall details later. Help arrange for follow-up care to lessen the emotional turmoil that the patient is experiencing.

Recognize the sexual problems associated with the reproductive process. Infertility, miscarriages, fetal anomalies, or death each present special problems. The patient and her mate need support as they work through their feelings.

Come to grips with your own beliefs and feelings about sexuality and sexual behavior. Reading and film attendance may be helpful. Separate your personal standards from those of the patient without being judgmental.

ORGANIZATIONS

1. American Association of Sex Educators and Counselors
2. Sex Information and Education Council of the U.S.
3. American Association of Marriage and Family Counselors
4. National Council on Family Relations
5. Reproductive Biology Research Foundation

The Patient with Somatic Complaints

Sometimes, when a patient's anxiety is so great that he cannot handle it effectively he displaces it onto parts of his body where it is felt as actual physical discomfort. One specific area of the body or several areas may be involved.

Perhaps the simplest illustration of a physical symptom caused by psychological factors is the tension headache. Commonly, one develops pain in the forehead, temples, and/or back of the neck and shoulders, which he associates with fatigue, tension, or worry. Characteristically, the pain is described as tightness, or "like a tight band." This feeling results from muscle contraction, which is the physical expression of emotional tension. The pain may be severe but can often be relieved by a mild analgesic. Eventually, the headache disappears without one ever really thinking through the reasons or events that precipitated it. One patient's severe headaches occurred during the morning hours, when the house physicians made their rounds. He was sure that he would be told his condition was deteriorating and that he would have to extend his stay in the hospital. The anticipation of such a finding had the physiological effect of producing severe tension headaches.

Physiological responses that are a reaction to a current situation are easily identifiable. Some patients, on observing others with more severe degrees of illness than they themselves have, are apt to identify and imagine that they have the same difficulties. They feel pains and discomforts in specific areas of the body, although no organic disturbance can be found. Later, when reassured that they do not have the more serious disease, the aches and pains disappear.

161

When an illness is diagnosed as psychosomatic in origin, the intimation is that the patient is reacting to earlier events that caused unconscious stress, and for which he is now showing physical symptoms. One patient complained of frequent migraine headaches over a period of five years. She was often so irritable that she lost various jobs and social relationships. Medication to relieve the throbbing helped, but not for long. Finally, she was referred for psychiatric care after a thorough neurological examination in the general hospital. When she was informed that no organic pathology for her headaches existed, she became upset and her complaints intensified as proof that she was being truthful. After many interviews, she was finally able to talk about a long-standing marital problem. Her husband had been seeing another woman for several years and while she didn't want him to leave, she could not tolerate the situation as it existed. She expressed her humiliation, resentment, and rage not only towards her husband, but towards herself. Until this time, she had not recognized that the conflict of intense hostility toward her husband, and her strong need and dependence on him, was being expressed in the form of a migraine headache. The patient was able to accept this interpretation more readily when told by the physician that the stress of her situation actually was causing the physiological changes that made her head throb.

A young college student was admitted to the hospital with severe headaches and tingling sensations in the arms and legs. She explained that these symptoms had existed for over a year, but now she felt they prevented her from continuing in school. The pain was intolerable. She had sought several medical opinions, but no organic reason for her discomfort had been uncovered. She was not hospitalized on the psychiatric unit but was seen in the general hospital for daily psychiatric interviews. During these interviews, the patient disclosed fear of being away at college, loneliness, inability to have meaningful friendships, lack of a boyfriend, and difficulty in achieving excellent grades. Initially, she was made aware of the tensions and anxieties that brought about the physiological changes which produced her symptoms. Since many tests were done, she felt that her symptoms were also important in themselves. As she expressed her feelings and attitudes toward the difficulties she was encountering, she revealed a deep underlying resentment towards an older brother. He was a very successful student, had an outgoing personality, and was, she felt, favored by their parents. Her inability to do as well in her studies as he did made her feel like a failure. Not being as popular as he was made her feel worthless. Her being away at school (despite the fact that this was her choice), while her brother was now at home, was interpreted as proof that her parents loved her brother more each day while rejecting her.

At this point, the patient was not aware that her symptoms were helping her to obtain attention from her parents and brother. At the same time, she had an acceptable reason for not doing as well as she thought she ought to in her work. Many weeks passed before she began to see that there was no reason for her to compete with her brother—that she was seen and liked by others for herself alone. Then she began to realize that she had to acknowledge and build her own strengths and work toward realistic, achievable goals instead of unobtainable ones. The expression of her feelings, and the acceptance of them, along with a great deal of staff support for the patient as she was, evoked a gradual subsidence of her symptoms.

The patient with a somatic complaint dwells on the ailment or discomfort and reports his symptoms to the staff repeatedly during the day. He seems to fear that unless he does so, no one will really believe him. He is concerned that if no real physical pathology is found, he will be labeled "crazy." As a result, some patients will go to great lengths to prove how incapacitated or uncomfortable they are—they moan and groan loudly, voice constant complaints, and request medication before the last dose has even begun to take effect. Citation of any improvement results in denial and is interpreted by the patient as a great injustice to him. He may even feel that the staff is trying to rob him of something quite precious and resolves that he is not going to give up without a big battle. In a sense, he is justified in feeling this way, especially if he does not have anything better with which to replace his physical symptoms.

Usually, patients with somatic complaints do not have demonstrable pathology; but some do, and then the physical sickness is actually triggered by emotional factors. This relationship has long been recognized. Just think of how the heart increases in rate and pounds in the chest when one experiences intense excitement such as meeting a lover or being in an automobile accident. Think of the intensity of gastrointestinal symptoms (nausea or diarrhea) that may occur when one anticipates taking an examination, giving a speech, or going to the analyst's office—all events that produce anxiety. The symptom manifested is the escape valve that relieves unbearable anxiety.

In the general hospital, the nurse cares for patients with ulcerative colitis, peptic ulcer, asthma, obesity, and hypertension. Although there is usually no doubt that actual physical changes which have adverse effects do exist in these patients, it is believed that emotional factors play a significant role in the course, and perhaps in the cause, of their physical illnesses. Flare-ups are common during periods of emotional stress. The patient will usually indicate that he feels "nervous" and "tense." However, he attributes the upset to his physical illness. One patient who survived several life-threatening bouts of ileitis told the staff that she would force herself to have an attack in order to get her husband to meed her demands. Occasionally, talking with the patient about how feelings and emotions cause illness can be therapeutic. But any long-term improvement in the condition demands long-term treatment. Recognition of this will decrease the feeling of ineptness one may experience when working with these patients, and increase one's tolerance and patience in a frustrating situation.

A patient with an acute illness such as myocardial infarction, cerebrovascular accident, or who has undergone gallbladder surgery has already sustained a jolt to his physical system and experienced much fear and anxiety. If his personality structure before illness was defective, the illness may be used manipulatively to escape difficult and unpleasant situations in the future. Thus, he may voice many complaints that are unrelated to the primary illness. This becomes especially apparent during convalescence, when the patient finds it threatening to recover completely. It is more satisfying to him to continue deriving the secondary gains that the illness has provided. These gains are seen in terms of extra attention, pity, a dependency relationship, and even disability insurance payments. An example of how this latter gain may be utilized was seen in the patient who was admitted to the hospital for long-standing neck pain. To offset the pain, he kept his head bent toward one side and, for years, this prevented him from working. He sought treatment only when his disability payments were discontinued. But, by this time his neck muscles on one side had become permanently shortened, and his condition was not amenable to treatment.

The patient admitted to a psychiatric unit for treatment of a psychically influenced somatic illness is incapacitated to the extent that his symptoms interfere with effective functioning. He hopes that psychiatric treatment will assist in alleviating his physical condition, which has been caused or intensified by tensions. He is told that if he can learn to deal with the emotional aspects of his life, his symptoms will decrease appreciably. This is often a difficult concept for the patient to accept. Thus, it is up to the staff to help him gain confidence and obtain some satisfaction in life that will replace his need for the symptom. This is no easy task. But the discomfort, unhappiness, and incapacity created by the patient's situation, plus his willingness to accept voluntary hospitalization, means that he recognizes the burden of his present predicament. He would like to make some changes, if only he could do so and at the same time save face.

An example of such a dichotomy is furnished by a young woman who was hospitalized because of severe anorexia. She had lost much weight, and her physical strength was deteriorating. Her behavior was related to deep hostility toward her mother, and was expressed by rejecting the food her mother prepared. This maladaptive pattern was corrected after much perseverance by the staff in trying to help the patient to see herself as worthy and meaningful, not just as an object who would not eat. No attempt was made to interpret the unconscious factors. The patient began to see how detrimental her behavior was to herself, and also that change was possible. As her good qualities were reinforced, her self-esteem improved, and successful treatment became possible.

In another case, a young woman in her twenties was admitted to the psychiatric unit because of a severe depression. She had made a suicidal attempt that was precipitated by a broken engagement. After admission, she developed pain in the legs and groin. She was unable to ambulate or stand erect. This persisted for two weeks, during which time a medical workup was completed in an effort to discover the source of her pain. Results of all tests were negative. She refused to discuss her engagement or other aspects of her personal life, and clung adamantly to her physical incapacity. In the course of many interviews, she revealed guilt regarding her sexual activity with the boyfriend and an incestuous relationship with an uncle when she was quite young. At this point, her physical complaints were explained to her as manifestations of the great anxiety she was experiencing regarding her sexual experiences. Her disappointment over the broken engagement and her embarrassment at telling family and friends revived the original repressed guilt related to her uncle. She unconsciously sought to avoid these aspects of her life which presented problems, and punished herself by developing symptoms in the body areas associated with sexual activity.

The patient cannot voluntarily control the symptom that develops in response to the stress of an earlier event. This is important for staff to keep in mind, as there is a tendency to regard the patient as being able to recover if only he would put his mind to it. This, of course, is not the case, as the patient is not able to view his condition with his conscious mind. The need for effective treatment and a supportive approach is intensified when the worker realizes that physiological symptoms which continue over long periods of time may result in unalterable body deformities.

THE APPROACH TO THE PATIENT
WITH SOMATIC COMPLAINTS

Evaluate the patient's complaint of physical pain. Do not be judgmental, even though the complaint does not appear to be valid. Inquire what was taking place when the patient first noticed the pain, and when and where it began. Express your willingness to understand what he is experiencing, without suggesting that it may be unreal. Remember that the patient's physical symptoms and his emotional problems influence each other. It may well be a sign of improvement if the patient's rash gets better or his diarrhea decreases.

Tell the patient that it must be very depressing to suffer as he does. He may then validate the existence of depression. It is difficult for most patients to admit that their pain is a result of a preceding depression. They prefer to believe the reverse, that the pain causes the depression. The patient with psychosomatic complaints has an absence of any organic findings. He often feels frustrated as his multitude of somatic complaints result in negative findings, baffling the health professionals. Patients with chronic complaints seek a reaction and a loving response from the health worker in the same way that a sick child seeks love from a parent. Unfortunately, their repetitive complaints drive away the people they need most. At the same time, the painful disorder satisfies an unconscious need for punishment.

Avoid giving well-meant but meaningless advice. Although you can suggest that some emotional problem may be increasing the patient's physical discomfort, avoid confrontation. Asking the patient what emotionally upsetting incident was going on when his ulcer first started is too direct a confrontation for the patient's defenses to handle and might prove disastrous. Stay away from such meaningless recommendations as, "Just learn to take things easy," "Relax," or "Don't be such a worrier." These suggestions accomplish nothing. Instead say, "I noticed you became upset when your mother visited you," or "I noticed you seemed upset when you didn't receive any mail this morning." This allows the patient to comment on real situations or problems that might be bothering him.

Let the patient talk about the physical aspects of his illness first. This will give you an understanding of his feelings about his illness, its cause, prognosis, and the limits it imposes. Try to discover which family members react to his illness, and how. Listen to what he has to say about how his life is affected or influenced, for better or worse, by the problem. Never underestimate the reasons why a person clings to his symptoms. The illness may be less of a problem for him than having to face his other difficulties. Discourage him from searching for shortcuts, such as a new pill or a different medical regime, since they are unlikely to have any lasting effect on his symptoms.

Encourage the patient to talk about things that have increased or decreased his aches and pains. Then help him to see that sometimes an upsetting telephone call can create a nervous reaction, resulting in diarrhea, headache, or other symptoms. Ask the patient, "What would you do if you were well?" Perhaps plans should be changed if the patient's illness is a way of avoiding his work, forthcoming marriage, moving to another state, engaging in sex, and so on.

Never reject, avoid, ignore or humiliate a patient because he has "no right" or "no cause to be sick." Never say, "The pains are all in your head." Accept him as he is and communicate the attitude that there is a reason for all illness. Say, "The staff will help you during your illness by working with you to understand yourself better."

Do not increase the patient's anxiety by telling him what seems obvious to you. If you say to the asthmatic, "Oh, I bet your hatred for your dead father is behind all this," you may well precipitate an attack. Do not attach a label to the patient or shake him off with an abrupt, "There is not one thing wrong with you. You're a perfectly healthy specimen." Patients who have somatic complaints use them for a purpose, whether to communicate with others or to protect themselves from unconscious fears. Encourage the patient to talk about times when the symptoms appeared. Tune in to periods in his history of loss, loneliness, disappointments, and dependency.

Encourage the patient to find small satisfactions and experience small achievements. This may allow him to feel secure enough to begin giving up his somatic complaints.

The Patient with Anorexia Nervosa

The news media have focused on anorectic patients during the past few years, leading many to believe that this disorder is peculiar to our times. In fact, it is an entity that was described as long ago as 1689, when the relationship between anorexia, constipation, amenorrhea, and overactivity was recognized. Although the condition is usually considered benign by lay people, fatalities were recorded as far back as 1789.

There are a variety of approaches that have been used in treating the anorectic patient. A purely somatic approach has been taken by some health professionals, increasing the caloric intake from 1,500 to 5,000 calories per day over a two-week period. If the patient refuses to eat willingly, the decision may be made to force feed her by means of tube feedings. In other instances, electrostimulative therapy has been used in an effort to produce an anabolic effect on the diencephalic centers of the brain. For some, hospitalization is ordered to separate the patient from her family. For others, family therapy on an outpatient basis is regarded as the treatment of choice. Behavior modification is another modality which may be utilized, giving permission for increased physical activity as a reward for weight gain. The fact that the approaches are so divergent is an indication that this is a very difficult disorder to treat.

Why should a patient (almost always an adolescent female) choose to starve herself when food is readily available? What kind of person would torture herself in this way? What kind of family would allow this to happen? Health professionals are often at a loss to understand the emaciated patient who forcefully states that nothing is wrong and who is uncomfortable if she gains a few ounces. Nor are they likely to recognize the distorted relationships between the patient and other family members. The patient may exhibit extremely antagonistic behavior to her relatives, yet will fight any attempt to remove her from the home, whether to a hospital, residential school, or other place. She clearly has difficulty in separating, particularly from her mother.

Anorectic patients arouse many negative feelings in care providers. Although the patient sees herself as being appealingly slim, she is more likely to be painfully emaciated. She looks like a skeleton covered with skin, with some ptosis of the abdomen. She often has rampant tooth decay, bluish mottling of her hands and feet, abnormally brittle nails, and very slight breast formation. One eighteen-year-old, who was five feet three inches tall and weighed seventy-six pounds, denied that she was underweight. The fact that she resembled a concentration camp victim, with her skeletal structure clearly visible under her skin, was not apparent to herself. However, regardless of her physical appearance, it is usually her behavior which alienates those who are trying to help. She is absolutely determined to maintain an emaciated state, denying that she is ill, even appearing somewhat euphoric about her ability to refuse food. She tends to have a very cold manner, an unchanging facial expression, and resists any attempts of the professionals to be friendly. She avoids sharing pertinent information about herself, rarely telling the whole truth about anything. She buys, collects, and stores an oversupply of items that she uses, such as shoes, underwear, linens, or household articles, yet does not use more than two or three of each. She needs the reassurance that things are available should they ever be needed.

Patients with anorexia nervosa often demonstrate an interest in food and its preparation. They collect recipes, cook, help with the serving and clean up. In these activities, they appear to emulate the mother/woman role. They will often appear panic stricken if the refrigerator or cupboards are not well stocked with food. Yet when food is served, they eat little, if anything. They manage to push the food around on their plates to give the appearance of having eaten. They also resort to hiding food in their napkins, discarding it in receptacles when unobserved, or eating well and then disappearing into the bathroom to stick their fingers down their throats and forcibly vomit whatever they have swallowed. They use laxatives and enemas as other ways of purging their bodies of food and exercise vigorously to lose weight.

It is important for health workers to realize that anorexia is only a *symptom* of a pathological state. The use of this particular symptom may be the patient's defense against more overt pathology, such as deep depression or suicidal thoughts. She may use starvation as a way to exert control over herself, her family, and her friends. To cure the symptom without treating the basic problem may well lead to an even more destructive behavior pattern.

Most patients with anorexia nervosa are described as having been very cooperative, pleasant, and highly disciplined during the premorbid phase. They tended to be involved only superficially with others, often fearful of new situations, but deeply entwined with family members. They did as they were told, dressed according to parental wishes, ate as much and as often as they were directed to, and went to bed or arose in accordance with the family rules. They never developed a sense of their own selves or had the opportunity to determine, among other things, whether or not they were hungry or satiated, hot or cold, sleepy or wide awake. If they did attempt to express some feeling, such as, "I'm very cold," it was likely to be invalidated by a comment noting, "You *can't* be cold. It's much too warm in here."

Often the anorectic behavior began the first time the child lived away from home, perhaps at a school or camp. Unable to recognize her satiation point, she continued eating as long as any food was available. In time, it became apparent that the only way to prevent overeating was not to eat at all. If she could not trust her own body to tell her when to stop, it was safer not to start.

In a society which emphasizes youth, beauty, and slender bodies, it is often mothers who coax their daughters to diet. The message, which is also stressed by the media, is that thin is preferable. Still compliant, the young, overweight adolescent begins to diet, and enjoys the praise that she receives from those around her. As time goes on, it becomes apparent to others that the degree of slenderness for which she strives is pathological, that her pursuit of thinness is an obsession as well as a compulsion. The individual's behavior about food changes radically. She refuses any plea to eat, appearing negative and obstinate. The stronger the command to eat, the more resistant the patient becomes, resorting to deceit and trickery if necessary so that she will appear to be eating even though she is not. The household begins to revolve around her.

The patient who is anorectic often recalls the teasing received as a youngster for her obesity, and blames her weight for rejection by friends. The more she was rejected or teased, the more she ate to ease the emotional pain. Although her mother may have appeared to be a caring person on the surface, doing whatever society deemed necessary in terms of household tasks, the history may reveal a lack of closeness between them. Food became a replacement for the missing emotional relationship; if the daughter ate, she accepted the "good" mother who prepared the food. The mother may have been ambivalent about her own role, absenting herself from the home because of work, recreation, or illness. On the other hand, she may have been a compulsive, rigid woman who forced her opinions on the family, demanding that the daughter do as she was told in every area of life.

Control is a very large issue in the life of an anorectic patient. She chooses self-starvation as her ultimate weapon, viewing it not as a self-destructive act, but rather as a way of controlling her own impulses. By not eating, she is making a statement. Even though she may crave food, she will not take it into her body. She alone is in total control of what will enter her body. She, rather than those around her (including her mother or the health care providers), is making the decision.

There are several other components at stake for the patient. Rejecting food, particularly that which has been prepared by her mother, is a covert way of rejecting her mother. The person who finds it difficult to develop an identity of her own within the family may not have the courage to separate from the other members. By rejecting the food provider's offering, she creates hostility in only one area of life. The family rallies around to get her to eat, yet their anger at her continuing use of starvation creates space between them and the patient. It is easier for the anorectic individual to deal with the family's hostility than to lose her hard-earned control over her own impulses.

Sexuality may be another issue for the patient. Most anorectic patients are adolescents who are uncomfortable with their new sexual awareness. They have never become sensitive to their other feelings, such as hunger or exhaustion, because their needs were met before they could be acknowledged. This new sexual sensation, for which they have not been programmed by mother, alarms them. If eating food may lead to a binge, then might a little sexual activity lead to promiscuity? Abstention is clearly the best course. Some adolescents fear pregnancy, equating it with an enlarged abdomen, and thus with eating. For them, self-starvation may be used as a contraceptive action to prevent oral impregnation. Once again, the patient sees herself to be in control of her sexual impulses, which she rejects as unacceptable. In addition, her anorectic state causes amenorrhea, and prevents breast development indicative of womanhood.

One patient recalled viewing her parents in the act of love-making when she was a young child. She heard her mother make sounds which she interpreted as groans of pain, and thought that her parents were doing "terrible and dirty things." She never talked about what she had seen. When her mother's subsequent pregnancy became noticeable, the patient associated it with the primal scene. She unconsciously feared that some man would do "dirty" things to her when she grew up. At the same time, she remembered her mother urging her to eat "so that you can be a mommy like me." Consequently, the patient stopped eating.

The parents of the anorectic patient frequently have a dysfunctional marriage. The patient may view each as having deficiencies and may feel responsible for providing sufficient attention to both to make up for their mutual deprivation. If the mother is away for a length of time, the daughter may be placed in the position of taking care of siblings and father. In one respect she delights in her pseudowifely role, for she can now give her father the understanding that he deserves. On the other hand, she resents being placed in the difficult position of acting as a parent to her siblings. She may have anticipated plaudits from her father for her efforts, but he may be too engrossed with responsibilities or concerns about his wife to offer recognition to the patient. He may repeatedly mention how much he misses his wife and how eager he is for her return. Moreover, the mother may not acknowledge her daughter's efforts either. The patient will see this as further proof that no one, not even a parent, is able to give her the affection and approval that she wants, even if she assumes a womanly role. Again, her anorexia will prevent her from developing or maintaining physical signs of womanhood, menstrual periods and breasts, which are present in her mother.

One hospitalized anorectic patient clearly demonstrated the cause and effect of family problems on the patient. She told of the two years her mother spent in a psychiatric hospital when the patient was five to seven years old. During visiting hours, the mother was too ill to talk to the daughter, which the child then assumed meant that her mother hated her.

The father was involved with the five other youngsters in the family and was unable to fill the patient's needs for affection and reassurance. The patient recalled that her father teased her and called her chubby at one point. Even though she was young, the patient was expected to assume some household duties and responsibilities for her younger siblings. She deeply resented this, but said nothing.

At the age of fourteen, the patient embarked on a self-imposed starvation diet and exercise program, which she was unable to recognize as a self-destructive weapon. She later said, "I felt this was the only way I could exercise some control over my life." The patient began therapy after medical advice had been sought for amenorrhea, hair loss, and her refusal to stop a fanatical exercise routine. Over several years of treatment, she recognized the relationship between her compulsion to be thin and her unconscious anger at her mother, her anger regarding home responsibilities, her need for affection and approval from her father, and her fear of growing up to be a woman like her mother.

Since many health workers are engaged in a personal battle against obesity, they may secretly admire the patient's adherence to a starvation regime. One overweight professional, on seeing the emaciated patient, said, "I'd like to have your illness for a few days." Attitudes such as these reinforce the patient's pathology and render the health worker ineffective in any treatment approach. In addition, the worker may not recognize the manipulative aspects of the patient's behavior, because he identifies with her. For example, the patient may complain relentlessly that she has not been able to defecate, and demand a laxative. The professional may accede to this request, not realizing that the laxative is being used to prevent any weight gain, rather than to treat constipation.

The anorectic patient reacts negatively to authority figures, since they represent the negative parent figure and threaten the control that the patient is exercising over herself. At times, the patient appears to cooperate, perhaps overeating ravenously, in order to make the health workers believe that she is cured. She will then return home and resume her chronic behavior very quickly. She has outsmarted the professionals, which lowers her regard for them and makes her feel that no one can really help her. She again has control of her body through her behavior.

Starvation is an effective fortification of the patient's precarious psychological balance and cannot be stopped for too long. When this symptom is taken away, she finds herself unable to control her other impulses. Having lost her control, she may demonstrate increased pathology, including suicidal behavior. In essence, the control, which she sees as absolute, is really quite tentative. It is an all-or-nothing situation—starvation or binge, with little hope for maintaining a middle road.

Often health workers assigned to anorectic patients resent the fact that they are cast into the role of law enforcement agents, having to check the patient's room and wastebasket for discarded food. They often voice anger that despite their own attempts to be helpful, the patient is unappreciative. The more effective they are, the more deceitful the patient becomes. Yet the involvement of a warm, supporting, and consistent health worker is essential in helping the patient establish her own identity.

Patients with anorexia nervosa object to hospitalization for good reason. An institutional setting encourages regression to a state of greater dependency, the very situation which they are fighting. However, there are times when the patient's physical state has deteriorated to such an extent that immediate medical intervention is required to maintain her life. She may require intravenous as well as tube feedings to supply sufficient fluid and nutrients. She will also need intensive psychotherapy to provide support as she is deprived of her most precious possession, her ability to control what goes into her body. One sixteen-year-old, enraged by her weight gain and the continuous supervision, proceeded to throw herself down a flight of stairs. Immediate intervention prevented any injury, but the patient announced that she intended to kill herself if necessary in order to escape from the restrictive hospital environment.

Family therapy is often used in order to change the emotional climate of the home environment. Improvement of the relationship between the parents, as well as between each parent and the patient, is necessary. The family may appear very resistant to this, offering a variety of excuses as to why they cannot institute any changes. If this occurs, it may be helpful to use a therapeutic paradox. To do this, the professional should insist that each family member, including the patient, continue using the same behavior patterns as before. The patient is once again placed in the position of being told what to do by an authority figure. Since control is the basic issue, she is likely to rebel by refusing to obey the order to continue her starvation pattern. To do this, she must give up her symptom and eat. The coalition of family against the professional's order is a healthy first step. Therapy with the family has to continue until the relationships are healthier, and the patient is recognized as an autonomous individual, capable of making decisions for herself.

THE APPROACH TO THE PATIENT WITH ANOREXIA NERVOSA

Encourage the patient to recognize her feelings about her body, including hunger, sleepiness, anxiety, etc.

Keep discussion of food and its intake to a minimum.

Make clear to the patient that responsibility and determination for her care is mainly under her control, rather than yours.

Encourage participation of the patient in her treatment by including foods she requests. Include other items which contribute to a well-balanced diet.

Do not become angry at the patient's deviant behavior, which may include spilling food on the floor, hiding food in her room, eating in binges, or forcing herself to vomit.

Explain to the patient that room checks may be necessary to validate whether food was eaten or hidden.

Give the patient choices in as many areas of her care as possible.

The patient should be confronted with her role in any weight loss while she is being treated. She may have been riding an exercise bike for several hours, doing vigorous calisthenics, or taking laxatives to lose weight.

Approach the patient several times daily to assure her of your personal interest. Be consistent when responding to her. (Anorectic patients tend to be manipulative, playing members who are inconsistent against one another.)

Be clear about your expectations of the patient. Make sure she knows that her participation in treatment is essential. Clear, consistent guidelines reinforce the patient's sense of self-control and increase her confidence in the health workers.

Give positive reinforcement when the patient cooperates.

Be aware of your feelings and responses to the patient. If the patient uses flattery in an effort to get a special privilege, calmly inform her that you recognize what she is doing. Do not react in an angry manner, since that would not be therapeutic.

Engage the patient in a relationship which emphasizes her value as a human being. If the patient can accept you as trustworthy and reliable, she will be more amenable to giving up her symptom on a permanent basis.

The Diabetic Patient

A middle-aged woman goes for a routine annual physical examination. During the course of reporting on how she has been all year, she mentions jestingly that she would really like to feel a bit more peppy, just in order to keep up with her teen-aged children. She states that sometimes she perspires too much and that she has lost weight even though she "eats like a horse." She attributes her weight loss to her active, independent life style. She mentions some minor inconveniences, such as having a small bladder which necessitates running to the bathroom frequently. But then she is always thirsty, so perhaps she should just stop drinking so much. It all sounds quite innocuous to her, but to the physician this attractive lady's complaints register immediately. Her attempts to make light of minor distresses demonstrate some anxiety. At the conclusion of a complete examination, which includes the necessary urinalysis and blood tests, a diagnosis of diabetes is established. When the patient is told this she smiles and displays a mixture of surprise and disbelief. Surely, there is an error. "Me, a diabetic?" The smile quickly gives way to serious concern as it is definitely established that no error has been made.

The health worker may first encounter the diabetic patient in the physician's office, during a hospital admission for another illness, or when there is an urgent admission for treatment of insulin shock or diabetic coma. What comes to mind is that this relatively common condition can become a rather severe management problem for many patients. Certainly the diabetic patient must adjust to changes in his living patterns. Fre-

179

quently, premorbid psychological patterns affect the way in which he does this as he tries to keep his illness under control. Sometimes the psychological problems may further aggravate the illness and thus interfere with its stabilization.

Many health workers believe that the more the patient knows and understands about diabetes, the more self-reliant and capable he will become in its management. Thus the patient is told that his body has a relative deficiency of the hormone insulin, which is necessary for the proper metabolism of glucose (sugar). This results in an inability of the body to make full use of food which has been ingested. When there is too much available and unutilized glucose in the body, it spills over into the urine and blood. To control the disease, the patient is given the missing substance (insulin), or an oral agent which stimulates insulin-producing cells. He is informed about a dietary regimen which regulates carbohydrate and caloric intake. He is taught how to test his urine for sugar and acetone. If insulin has been ordered, he is taught how to inject it himself.

This all sounds easy. What makes for complications is that often the patient's problems, including premorbid ones, as well as his attitudes and outlook, may adversely affect his ability to make the adjustments necessary for living with his illness.

The health worker frequently encounters a diabetic who denies having the illness; he simply refuses to accept the diagnosis. He sets out to prove that he is the master of his own body, always in control. He will allow nothing to direct his life, nor will he submit himself to a ridiculous regimen of injections. He will not be humiliated, lose self-esteem, or be known in any way, shape, or form as someone with a health problem. He refuses to learn to inject himself and fails to stay on any semblance of a diet. He refuses to believe that the consequences of uncontrolled diabetes may be life-threatening.

Such was the case of a forty-two-year-old successful business woman and mother of five. She was a very active and forceful person. In her job she had considerable influence and control over others. In her home she was the main provider and dominating partner. In the hospital she was unresponsive and resistant to any teaching or discussion of her disease. Even though the staff emphasized the fact that she would eventually be able to regulate her insulin dosage and diet, she refused to acknowledge or cooperate with the therapeutic regimen set up for her. Needless to say, this presented a serious problem for the patient, since her diabetes could not be regulated. The staff felt futile and ineffective at first, and then hostile towards the patient for her uncooperative behavior, which resulted in several brushes with death.

The individual who is basically dependent also presents problems. He may regress further, and refuse to have any part in the management or control of his illness. He first becomes immobilized by his disease, and then finds that being cared for meets a deep need, and therefore is a pleasurable prospect. The fact that he has diabetes may even serve to increase his anxiety, which in turn increases his need to be dependent. He may therefore exhibit a helplessness which demands that everything be done for him. When his needs are not met, he may lapse into apathy and depression.

The adult diabetic who is depressed may act on his desire to end his life by going off his diet or neglecting to take his insulin. Or, if the patient feels he is being punished for his misdeeds through his illness, he may become hostile and resentful. He may express his anger and frustration by overeating.

Emotional conflicts and reactions are often activated by the diabetic patient's dietary restrictions. The psychological significance of food is related to support, love, and acceptance. When denied certain foods, the patient may have increased feelings of being unloved, rejected, unwanted. This can pose particular problems in the already obese individual who overeats to satisfy frustrated drives and to increase his feeling of well-being. The reverse situation is seen in the patient who is unable to eat, or refuses to, when he becomes upset. "You make me unhappy so I just won't eat," is what is unconsciously meant. This behavior may cause a hypoglycemic reaction.

Young diabetics may use the disorder as a way of controlling their parents by threatening to disregard their dietary regimen if their request for a new car, for an increase in allowance, or for new clothes is not granted. They may express their anger by undereating, overeating, or failing to take their insulin. Parents themselves may unconsciously resent the trouble or be unable to deal with the guilt of having a diabetic youngster.

As a result, they may be either too rigid or too lax in their attention to the child's diet. Youngsters then use the diabetic condition to manipulate them.

Youngsters are often resistant to limitations placed on them by the disorder. If denial is strong, the patient may attempt to prove he can eat anything he desires. This sets the stage for a severe hyperglycemic reaction necessitating hospitalization. Diabetic youngsters often feel that because they are not like everyone else, they aren't worth loving. Special attention and cooperation from parents are essential.

In one case, a nineteen-year-old female was admitted to the intensive care unit in a diabetic coma. During recovery, she related that she had had an argument with her parents, who objected strenuously to her dating a boy of dubious character. They had threatened to withhold funds they had promised to help finance her education. She was furious that they did not realize how seriously she felt about her boyfriend, and wanted to punish them for not viewing the relationship as she did. She expressed her anger by omitting her insulin and by ingesting several frankfurters, some candy, and a malted milk shake. Her diabetic reaction almost cost her her life.

The health worker must be aware of certain very real and irksome inconveniences that the diabetic faces. Emotional stress may raise his blood glucose level. (In fact, the onset of the disease is itself often related to a stressful period in the patient's life.) When under stress, the patient may develop such psychological symptoms as increased sensitivity, fright, or forgetfulness. He should be encouraged to talk about these feelings and experiences. The health worker can then help him to seek new ways of managing stressful problems before they arise.

The diabetic patient often needs help in seeking and obtaining wholesome satisfactions and pleasures to offset those he is denied. Practicing self-denial is difficult for anyone, so imagine what it is like for the diabetic, who must do this on a continual basis. He also has to learn to deal with feelings of awkwardness or embarrassment if he has to take insulin while on the job, before a social event, or when on a trip. He may have to increase his intake of glucose when participating in sports, and he must be able to test his urine frequently. He is apt to fatigue easily and then develops a sense of frustration when his lack of energy prevents him from doing or accomplishing all he desires. Sometimes this leads him to ignore the whole regimen, and test his limits. Female patients often feel unfeminine and unattractive because they perspire heavily. The patient's self-image may thus be impaired, and she may blame her inability to attract men, obtain employment, or have friends on the illness.

Whether the diabetic makes a successful adjustment to his illness may depend on the successful working-through of emotional conflicts that existed before the illness and that are now aggravated by it. Concerns regarding future illnesses, fears of becoming incapacitated, doubts about the advisability of having a baby, and worries about dying can be activated. The special meaning of illness must be explored with each and every diabetic patient. The special problems and fears encountered by each patient must be clarified. The health worker should take as much time as needed to uncover the feelings aroused by the illness, as well as their conscious and unconscious implications. The patient needs all the support he can get if he is to make a satisfactory adjustment to living with his condition.

THE APPROACH TO THE DIABETIC PATIENT

Encourage the diabetic patient to talk about his fears, feelings, problems. Recognize that his denial of illness is a manifestation of an emotional conflict. Do not react angrily or reprimand him. Instead tell him, "I understand how upset you must be. Other patients have learned to manage successfully with treatment and, in time, you will also." Explain to the patient that it is important to deal with what exists, even though at times it is painful. Assure him that he will be given every assistance in learning new ways of living. Be aware that the patient's moodiness, fright, or forgetfulness may be related to an unregulated glucose level.

Be empathetic in regard to the difficulties and hardships the patient encounters in controlling his illness. But stress his rewards and gains in doing so. Maintain an optimistic attitude. Recognize the fact that the patient can continue to lead his usual adequate and constructive life.

Emphasize the individual's strengths and independent abilities. Allow the patient to do all he can for himself, even though it may seem easier to do things for him. Minimize his dependencies. Instruct him about anything that will make his life easier. Inform him about how to protect his clothing from perspiration odor by wearing absorbent, loose garments, about the use of special soaps that will help prevent infection, and about how to cut his toenails and care for his feet correctly.

Understand that a patient with diabetes can be a real suicidal risk. The patient may act out his desire to die by not taking insulin or by over-eating. Attempt to persuade him to seek relief from his hostility and frustration through acceptable channels. He can take a brisk walk, involve himself in group activities, punch a punching bag, or pound a pillow.

Do not argue with the patient regarding his noncompliance or lack of cooperation. Instead, point out that his behavior is related to an upsetting incident in his life, perhaps precipitated by an argument. Tell him, "It appears that everytime your girlfriend and you argue, you overeat," or "It appears that your worry about your work causes you to forget to eat on a regular basis." In other words, help the patient to connect his behavior with the problem that caused it. Then help him develop a plan for new ways of reacting to and handling his problems.

Encourage the young diabetic to test his own urine and give himself insulin as soon as possible. The more the youngster can do for himself, the less restricted he will feel.

The Patient with a Mastectomy

Cancer of the breast is the most common form of cancer in women. Between 5 and 10 percent of women in the United States can be expected to develop breast cancer. Some women discover for themselves that they have a lump in one of their breasts. Others are unaware of the presence of a lump until it is found on routine physical examination. The reaction to a lump in a breast is often a combination of denial and fear. "No, not me; it just can't be," is the common reaction. Often, the woman waits through the next menstrual cycle in the hope that the lump will disappear. If it has been discovered by a physician, the patient may seek another consultation, hoping for a different finding, one that will result in the statement, "It's okay, you don't need to have the operation."

The possibility of a mastectomy is a frightening prospect. Before this procedure is carried out, a biopsy is done to determine whether or not the lump is cancerous. If it is noncancerous (benign), only the area of the growth is removed, the incision is stitched, and no more need be done. Needless to say, this patient is relieved of much anxiety and fear. But if the mass is cancerous (malignant), then the entire breast, including even uninvolved breast tissue, plus the surrounding axillary nodes and lymphatic vessels may be excised in the hope of removing any and all unseen spreading cancer cells. This surgical procedure is known as radical mastectomy. Some surgeons prefer to perform modifications of this procedure. However, the decision as to the type of surgery will depend on the stage of the cancer and the judgment of the surgeon.

It is not unusual for a woman to give permission solely for a biopsy.

If further surgery is needed, she will then have additional time to prepare herself psychologically and to discuss with her physician the kind of surgery she will undergo. This is a controversial action, since a positive biopsy means that the woman will subject herself to anaesthesia twice and will also risk the possibility of disseminating the tumor if cells from the biopsy area escape into her blood stream. Nevertheless, more and more women are opting for a decided role in determining what, if any, treatment should be employed.

The breast is a primary sex symbol in our culture. The breasts have become a source of admiration, overemphasized to the point that they have been equated with a woman's sexual desire, sexual drive, desirability, and even sexual competence. The notion that men are primarily attracted to a female's breasts has also been propagated. Thus, many women have come to believe that the removal of a breast will make one less desirable, less sexual, and less feminine. Believing this, it is no wonder that patients who undergo a radical mastectomy fear they will be rejected by their friends and unloved by their spouses. In their own eyes, they appear irreparably damaged.

The deformity created by a mastectomy is greatly feared. A woman may feel repulsed by the sight of her incisional scar and be unable to make love freely. She does not want anyone to see her body, and even spares her spouse the sight. If she does resume sexual activity, she may never again remove her brassiere or prosthesis. Thus, even the remaining breast is withdrawn from the fondling lover. Self-consciousness may become so strong that the patient wears only clothing that covers her neck and arms, and will not wear a bathing suit, because she is sure that everyone on the beach is staring at her.

Additional difficulties involve shopping for clothes, especially in stores where individual dressing rooms may not be available, or where an eager salesperson may increase the risk of the patient's deformity being noticed. On the other hand, some clothing manufacturers are now meeting the needs of mastectomy patients with well-fitting, attractive clothes that hide unsightly scars. Unfortunately, many women avoid resumption of sports activities or being in places that include large groups of people because they fear accidental injury to the remaining breast, as well as the possibility of rejection.

If a woman is of childbearing age, special significance may be attached to the inability to breast-feed a child. The patient may feel that she is not a fit mother because the child cannot be cuddled to the breast. If she has passed the childbearing age, she may have feelings of inadequacy as a mother and verbalize feelings of guilt because she did not breast-feed when she could have given the baby this supposed advantage. On occasion, the child that has been breast-fed has been blamed by the woman as being the cause of the cancer because she remembers that he suckled or bit down too hard.

Some women have built their total life and self-value on good looks and a great body, without developing their other assets. In other words, they lack a true sense of self. They have emphasized looks, and have judged others by this value to such a degree that they are unable to see that there is more to life than physical appearance. They cannot accept the fact that there are people in the world who build friendships on good faith, understanding, and mutual interest, for better or worse. These women need a great deal of help in reassessing their values. They need to develop other aspects of their individuality in order to build self-confidence. They need to experience acceptance, interest, and friendship, for themselves rather than for their appearance. This will take time because usually these individuals doubt that other people sincerely like them or want an association with a not-quite-whole person. This is because they have not yet accepted themselves as really worthy.

Regardless of how prepared a woman is for a mastectomy, anxiety, depression, and concerns about sexuality are almost always experienced. The patient has to adjust to coping with the loss of a breast, and will be reminded of her loss every day as she bathes, looks in the mirror, shops for clothes, or makes love. Additionally, she has to adjust to knowing that she has cancer, and the implication of what this means in terms of her future comfort and life span. The worry about the possible spread of the disease, loss of the other breast, or metastasis to other areas of her body is ever-present.

Some patients in the hospital are overly cheerful and appear to be making a great adjustment to their condition. "She's handling everything so well," health workers observe, secretly relieved that all discussion about the surgery can be avoided. This is in contrast to others, who are so overwhelmed with sadness that they are unable to talk. The cheerful patient may become depressed after leaving the hospital environment, when she is alone with the reality of her situation. The patient who has been depressed in the hospital will usually sink deeper into despair, withdrawing from all social contacts and rejecting the attempts of family members to be helpful. Since both patients have similar needs, it behooves the health worker to assume an approach of active inquiry into the patient's emotional state.

"How do you feel today?" is usually interpreted by the patient as referring solely to her physical problems and is answered on that level with, "My pain is less," or "My dressing seems dry." This leaves the emotional aspects untreated. It is important for the health worker to pause, pull up a chair, and encourage the patient to share her feelings, stresses, and distresses. The use of questions which are open-ended are more conducive to eliciting a discussion of problems. For example, "What kind of thoughts are you having about yourself?" or "How are you getting yourself ready for discharge?" are more apt to let the patient know that the health worker wants to share her burdens and is really concerned and interested in the difficulties she faces.

Many patients express the realistic concerns about the high price of prosthetic breast devices and the refusal of insurance companies to consider them as a medically valid expense. In fact, a woman's need to feel psychologically as well as physically whole is important. Loss of employment because of a mastectomy is another area which presents problems, particularly in light of heavy medical expenses and the need for the patient to be involved in worthwhile activities. Although job loss is discriminatory and therefore contrary to human rights laws, it may be impossible for a woman to continue working if the demands of work and home responsibilities result in extreme fatigue, particularly if chemotherapy or radiation therapy is required. If the patient is a divorced or widowed mother, she will be concerned about rearing her children, and about their care if she is no longer able to do so.

Involving the spouse in the care of his wife is of utmost importance, since the patient is very vulnerable to the possibility that she will be unloved or that her spouse will turn away from her in disgust. The help of an aware, knowledgeable, understanding husband can be a vital asset to a patient during an exceedingly stressful time. The husband, if at all possible, should go with his wife to all appointments to the surgeon, radiologist, and oncologist. He should be included in all discussions regarding his wife's care. He should know that if the biopsy is malignant, a mastectomy will be done. His thoughts and feelings should be elicited repeatedly. After all, this is also a stressful and frightening time for him. He has to keep himself together, support his wife emotionally, and sustain the family. Discussion about expected postoperative reactions such as anxieties and depressive reactions is helpful.

Some husbands experience an adverse reaction to their wives' operations because it brings a fear of being mutilated to the conscious mind. This is associated with the male fear of castration, and may result in rejection of the wife, who already feels that she is unappealing. The rejection is often really the spouse's reaction to his own fears and feelings, symbolized by the wife's operation.

If a marriage is already in trouble, the spouse may view surgery with satisfaction because it serves as a release for his anger. Other men may interpret the wife's surgery as a form of punishment for all the wrongs she has inflicted on him. Some men have never matured, and when they married did so because of the extra notice they would receive from others because of this new acquisition. If the wife was just another status symbol to show off to others or to make other men jealous and envious, then the husband may now believe that others will think he is stuck with a worthless, inadequate, and undesirable person. In truth, he thinks only of himself, not of his mate.

Many men do not understand what to do, what to say, or how to behave during the wife's readjustment period. Should he act as if nothing has happened? Should he pamper her? Should he cancel all social obligations? Should he continue love-making? Should he avoid looking at her when they are dressing? Will the wife be an invalid? Will their life style change?

A spouse who reinforces the idea that he married his wife for more than her breasts, while at the same time demonstrating compassion for her loss, can have a significantly positive effect in the patient's recovery. The husband who sees the operative area (a major hurdle for both spouse and patient) while in the hospital can dispel many conscious and unconscious fears. He should also be encouraged to help with his wife's care at home, by changing dressings, massaging the arm on the affected side, and helping with exercises. The husband should be strongly encouraged to initiate sexual intercourse unless his wife is too debilitated or clearly rejects any sexual contact. The persistent spouse who overtly demonstrates his sexual interests in his wife clearly gives her the message that he still finds her sexually attractive, exciting, and feminine. The spouse should be instructed to use sexual positions that provide the least upper trunk pressure (usually male superior). Patients will usually avoid the female superior position, although it avoids any upper torso contact, because it emphasizes the absence of the breast.

The husband should not pressure his wife to undress in front of him, or insist on nudity. Importance should be placed on sharing the heavy load of emotional feelings, reinforcing the wife's feelings that she is still loved, and encouraging an optimistic attitude about their future together. For many couples, the sharing of this traumatic and emotional experience deepens their value of life in general and their relationship in particular.

The fear and feelings of the patient, both before and after surgery, are usually related to her memories of past experiences. If the woman's childhood and adulthood were healthy and she developed a positive feeling about herself, then she will be able to love herself despite her loss. The family's way of viewing life, as well as their attitude toward the patient, is a significant factor in recovery. Often, the patient's response is related to an ongoing family problem, rather than the immediate surgical situation.

Inability to accept the gravity and urgency of the situation may be recognized in women who delay seeking medical attention, despite the fact that they know there is a growth in the breast. One patient who delayed the operation related experiencing a tremendous sense of relief when it was finally over. She felt she could now move forward, and begin to plan her life, whereas before she was immobilized by doubts, indecision, and fear. More dramatic is the refusal of some women to accept surgery despite the physician's urgent recommendations. The nurse then must provide a great deal of understanding, and emphasize the threat to the patient's life while stressing the potential life-saving results of surgery.

Following surgery, a patient's lack of cooperation as well as her overt anger may very well mean that she was ill prepared for the surgery that occurred. Some patients appear either unwilling or disinterested in learning how to rehabilitate themselves. They seem unmotivated, and remain apathetic about learning to care for the incision or going to available exercise classes. They do not want to discuss breast prostheses and refuse to talk with someone who has fully recovered from a similar experience. These patients demonstrate the involvement of the emotions in this type of surgery, and are actually attempting to deny the reality of their situation.

Many women are pleased with the new prosthetic breasts that are available, and some are even fitted before discharge from the hospital. However, many women are turning to reconstruction therapy for restoration or augmentation of the removed breast. This is prompted by a woman's desire to feel physically attractive, whole, and feminine. To a lesser extent it is prompted by dissatisfaction with the prostheses, and the problems created when the bra frequently moves up on the affected side. There is considerable controversy regarding the safety of implants, including the possibility that they may prevent detection of disease, or even cause disease. Some patients are psychologically helped if a consultation with a plastic surgeon is done before surgery, so that they can be assured that enough skin and muscle will be available for breast reconstruction. This can lead to disappointment if the size and spread of the tumor precludes the possibility of future reconstruction. This is often the situation if axillary node involvement is present. A waiting period of at least two to three years is often advised before undertaking reconstructive surgery. However, other surgeons believe that immediate reconstruction is advisable to lessen the emotional trauma to which the patient is subjected.

The nurse must take an active part in teaching and clarifying information. For example, many patients do not know that the breast is not essential for menstruation and hormone production. They need to know that following cessation of lactation, when the breasts cease to provide nutrition for the infant, they often become flat, less firm, and functionless. They need to know that prosthetic devices can be bought which make the body appear symmetrical. They need to be reassured that their previous life style need not be altered. They need to know and feel that they are still themselves. The nurse who sees mastectomy as unacceptable to herself, or finds herself unconvinced that full recovery is possible or that the patient can live a full life, will do well to examine her own sense of values and her own self image. For, surely, if she has difficulty in this area she will not be able to help the patient effectively.

A final word regarding the patient with breast cancer that has spread to the axillary lymph nodes and the adjacent tissues. Despite radical mastectomy followed by cobalt treatment, many women experience recurrence of overt disease. Often the nurse will become upset because it appears that the patient never talks about the operation and the current ongoing treatment. For example, one patient, the mother of eight children, seemed to be avoiding and denying the entire situation, making the nurse uncomfortable with what she felt was the patient's "sick" approach to life. The woman talked about plans for redoing her kitchen, planned dinner menus, looked forward to the imminent birth of her daughter's baby, and happily anticipated the growth of her sons to manhood when they would be able to fend for themselves. She did not dwell on her illness, nor on her prognosis. Her endurance and persistence were most admirable. It was important for the nurse in this instance to recognize the value of denial in terms of what the patient faced, rather than viewing the behavior as a sign of psychic illness.

THE APPROACH TO THE PATIENT
WITH A MASTECTOMY

Make yourself available to talk with the patient about her feelings. Acknowledge the loss. Say to the patient, "This must be a very difficult time for you." This allows the patient to tell you more about her difficulty. Gear the conversation to the patient as she is now. Do not dwell on the loss of her breast. Do not say, "Don't worry, everything will be all right," or "No one will ever know you wear a false one." This just skirts the subject and stifles further communication. Instead say, "As you begin to recover, you will gradually feel better. As you are able to do a little more each day, you will be reassured. Then we can begin to talk about the cosmetic breast prostheses that are available and that hundreds of women use." Clarify the patient's misconceptions about sexual matters, breast function, future activities.

Stress the way you are going to help the patient by:
1. Being with her on her return from the recovery room;
2. Having medication available to alleviate her pain;
3. Ambulating her as early as possible;

4. Supporting and elevating the affected arm; and
5. Beginning the prescribed exercises, and gradually increasing them in order to restore full range of motion in the affected arm.

Prepare the patient preoperatively for what to expect. No patient should wake up from surgery and find her breast removed without having been told that a frozen section of the biopsy, done at the time of surgery and studied by a pathologist, will determine if the breast must be removed.

Do not force a patient to do more than she is able. Support the patient if she is unable to view the operative area or insists on wearing her bra all the time. It is more important for the patient to feel that she is understood than for her to meet a timetable in acceptance of her physical loss.

Build on the patient's past accomplishments and strengths. If the patient is a mother talk about her involvement in that role; if a professional, help her plan her future. Encourage her to return to work as soon as possible so as not to lose her skills.

Compliment the patient for her effort and motivation and for her interest in doing for herself. Let her know that she is still looked upon as an attractive person.

Put the emphasis on life ahead. Stress the future. If the patient refuses surgery, emphasize, "Your life can be more normal if the doctor proceeds with the operation at this time." Try to get the patient to see that her life is not ending because of the mastectomy, but that a new life is beginning for her.

Talk with the husband. Elicit and assess his reaction to the surgery. What are his feelings? What is the state of his relationship with his wife? What special meaning does this operation have for him? Does he have any preconceived ideas about what his behavior should be? One husband stopped making love to his wife because he thought she would not want to participate. She, however, felt that his behavior indicated that he found her unsightly. She felt unwanted and neglected, not realizing that he thought he was being considerate. Remember, an informed, understanding, compassionate spouse gives true aid during a woman's recovery.

Recognize the symptoms of depression and approach the patient consistently. If a patient continues to grieve and says, "My life can never be the same; it's all over," assess the suicidal risk and the need for immediate intervention. The nurse should convey her belief in a hopeful outcome. She must work through her feelings in relation to her own reaction to breast cancer. Although the patient may be reluctant to look at herself, and may anticipate a disintegration of her life style, her fear of future illness and of possible death are really her main concerns.

Recognize the right of the patient to use denial as an asset in helping her to function each day.

The Patient
with Coronary Heart Disease

The leading cause of death in this country is cardiovascular disease, with coronary heart disease accounting for more than 50 percent of these deaths. No wonder then that the patient's reaction is one of overwhelming fear when he realizes that his heart is affected, particularly if the damage interferes with its adequate functioning.

Although many types of heart disease are serious, this chapter deals mainly with the condition of acute myocardial infarction. In this condition, a portion of the heart (myocardium) is destroyed because of an insufficient supply of blood to the affected area. This occurs when one of the coronary arteries which supply blood to the heart muscle, is closed or blocked in any way. The sudden onset of this life-threatening illness presents a major crisis to the individual, who previously may have appeared well. He suddenly experiences symptoms which may include severe weakness, excruciating chest pain, rapid pulse, a drop in blood pressure, and profuse sweating. He is aware that something is drastically wrong, and feels an urgent need for help. Life in all its many aspects has been interrupted without warning, and all the patient's thoughts and energies are directed to the process of survival. This is so basic that it is imperative for the staff to realize what this aspect of the illness means to a patient, what some of his possible emotional reactions are, and what psychological factors are important in helping him towards recovery.

During this initial stage of his illness, the patient may be cared for in a regular hospital unit or in a special unit for coronary care. Usually, he is terrified that he may die. The seriousness of the immediate situation is reinforced by his enforced immobilization, the administration of oxygen and possibly intravenous fluids, and the special medication that is given to help regulate his heartbeat. Constant monitoring on the oscilloscope, with his electrocardiogram observable at all times, adds to the patient's sense of impending doom. This, too, is understandable since he may have difficulty breathing and may be experiencing pain. Again, these difficulties may be magnified by the environment with its elaborate equipment, beepers, and monitors. Often the personnel present a somber appearance as they go about their work. The patient in a cardiac unit may possibly witness the cardiac resuscitation and defibrillation of another patient lying close by. He may also witness a death, since one in ten patients with coronary heart disease will die.

Being a coronary patient brings about a drastic change in the individual's routine of daily living. A healthy, independent personality suddenly feels helpless and dependent. This is somewhat reinforced by the patient's isolation from friends and family, and his need to rely on total strangers who know little about him personally. Furthermore, all his activities are restricted, communication via telephone is denied, and visits with friends or relatives are limited to brief periods. The patient is often fed by others and not allowed to bathe or shave himself. He is told not to lift, turn, or in any way strain himself. Through all this, he is told, ironically, that he must not worry or upset himself. "Let us do the worrying and doing" is a remark commonly heard and easier said than done, for the patient's mind is active. He is bombarded by a multitude of thoughts that center on his fears and anxieties.

Patient care in the coronary unit focuses on immediate attention to life-threatening situations which may arise at any instant. The nurse is the one in contact with the patient day and night. She makes every effort to keep him as comfortable as possible, while maintaining his vital functions at normal or near normal levels. Much of her effort is preventive. Throughout all this, the patient feels keenly the seriousness of the care being given to him.

The medical-surgical nurse in this setting must be thoroughly familiar with the unit's protocol and routine. She must keep the crises manageable. She must be a capable observer of physical signs, i.e., blood pressure, heart rate, pulse quality and rate, urine volume per unit time, warmth or coldness of the skin, diaphoresis, color, respiratory rate and quality. She must be well versed in the use of cardiac monitoring equipment, cardio-verters, defibrillators, and pacemakers. She must be familiar with the procedure of checking central venous pressure and other body-pene-trating lines. Indeed, as with most other disciplines, the more one knows, the better.

Often, the nurse is the patient's first contact on arrival at the hospi-tal. The rapport and confidence she establishes initially will serve the patient well during his difficult days of acute illness. It is during the first few days, especially the first and second, that the patient's anxiety and fear are at their height, and must be dealt with by the nurse. Symptoms of anxiety include pain, rigidity, tremors, sweating, restlessness, excessive talkativeness, insomnia, agitation, and weakness. It follows that keeping the anxiety level down is most beneficial to the patient.

The anxiety of a patient can be so high that he is unable to concen-trate on or retain explanations regarding care and procedures. Frequent repetition in the days that follow is needed to impart knowledge, reduce anxiety regarding procedures (especially the monitor alarm system), and encourage confidence and trust. Reducing fear is a primary task, as it may be a determinant in escalation of a mild ischemia to a fatal arrhythmia. Medication such as morphine may be used in this case not only to alleviate pain but also to reduce anxiety. If a patient should experience cardiac arrest and survive, it goes without saying that the health professional must help the patient talk about his feelings in order to help him accept the experience.

Depression is a common occurence during the third and fourth days. The patient manifests a sad and hopeless mood and is very pessimistic. He may weep because he feels that since he is physically unsound, and inac-tive, he is therefore useless. He may begin to verbalize anger by making sarcastic remarks and being critical of the nurse and the way the hospital operates. He may ask "Why me?" In his anger he may refuse to follow the nurse's suggestions. Some patients may have avoided responsibility as often as possible when they were well. Now the illness provides a second-ary gain in the form of permanent relief from obligations. Such a person may develop into what is commonly known as a "cardiac cripple." In con-trast, the patient who has had a dynamic, outgoing personality may be unable to face his illness with its threat of future loss, restriction of activities, possible reduction in income, change in his occupation or even in such pleasant habits as smoking and eating. He may deny that he ever had a heart attack and threaten to sign out of the hospital, stating that there is really nothing wrong with him. Still another patient may react to his illness by becoming overly cheerful. He takes everything the worker says lightly, attaches little importance to restrictions, and has a good word for everyone with whom he comes into contact. This patient's behavior indicates that he is not accepting the experience for what it is.

In an effort to ward off depression, the patient may become angry and verbalize his annoyances. Expressions of anger often give the patient the feeling of being in control as well as a feeling of exhilaration. Patients sometimes attempt to fight depression by clinging to the health professional, who provides continuous care. This helpless dependency is similar to a child who must have his parent to protect him from the mysterious outside world. The use of antidepressant medication requires prudence and alertness to possible adverse side effects such as tachycardia or palpitations. By the same token, cardiovascular disease may be treated with drugs that inadvertently precipitate depression.

The male patient who fears that his illness may cause the loss of his sexual prowess may make suggestive remarks to the nurse, comment on her figure, or openly invite her to have sex with him. He may tell off-color jokes and stories at every opportunity. This behavior can be attributed to denial as well as an attempt to cover up his uncomfortable depressed feelings by using the quick satisfaction of pleasant sexual thoughts.

It behooves the nurse to bear in mind that adjustment to a completely new way of life is difficult for all patients, and impossible for some. A patient may pass the critical period of his illness, begin to feel better quickly, and then be unable or unwilling to follow instructions that limit his way of life. In anticipation of possible refusal by the patient to accept limitations, the nurse will do well to learn all she can about his family, occupation, habits, and idiosyncrasies. This will enable her to plan an approach that is not only in the patient's best interest, but one that is also meaningful and suited to his total personality.

The nurse will be the one in most frequent contact with the family. She must understand their confusion, anxiety, and fear of approaching the patient. The hurried rush to the hospital, the urgent admission procedures, and then seeing the patient with his many alarming attachments frightens and oftimes bewilders his relatives. The nurse can have a positive influence on the visitors by her calm demeanor and the intelligent explanations she offers. She should provide time for the family to talk about their feelings, a need that cannot be overemphasized. By communicating with the family, the nurse obtains information regarding the personal life and habits of the patient. At the same time, she may serve as a sounding board for the family to work through some of their own fears, apprehensions, guilt, and anger. The nurse should observe the effect of family members on the patient, and deal with any expressed feelings which may adversely affect him by complicating his course of recovery. Family support for the patient may determine whether the treatment is a success or failure.

The nurse who cares for the coronary patient must be sensitive to her own behavior and reactions. Does she handle herself with ease, or is she always in a state of rush or uncertainty? Does she speak distinctly, calmly, and with confidence, or is she tense and vague while mumbling her words? Does she react defensively to the patient's anger and criticism, or does she recognize it as his reaction to his illness? Is she flexible and able to meet the patient's changing needs, or does she always unconsciously strive to satisfy her own needs? The patient observes how anxious the nurse is about his condition, and comes to his own conclusion about the seriousness of his illness.

Staff members go through a myriad of responses, such as depression, anxiety, cooperation, or hostility. It is not unusual to see the staff work together in tense unison while attempting resuscitative measures, only to lapse into a sullen mood after their efforts have failed. Staff members are not immune to displacement of angry feelings onto one another in an attempt to ward off depressive reactions when a patient dies or is ill beyond their ability to help.

THE APPROACH TO THE PATIENT
WITH CORONARY HEART DISEASE

Be truthful. Give the patient honest and clear answers. Remember, he is usually alert, aware of everything you are doing, and frightened. Respect his intelligence. It is better to acknowledge to him that his illness is serious than to pretend that it's not. The patient will assess your answers and make his own decision as to whether he can rely on you for an honest answer in the future. This will undoubtedly influence your relationship with him.

Assure the patient that measures are being taken to keep him as comfortable as possible. Let him know that the medical and nursing team has everything under control. Mention, "Your breathing will be much easier as you breathe the oxygen and after you receive this medication." Always tell the patient what you are doing to help him. Make sure he understands the unpleasant restrictions that have been ordered—a special diet, limited visitors, and bed rest. These should be explained with emphasis on their helping qualities. "We are enforcing the doctor's orders vigorously because we want you to recover as quickly as possible."

Allow several periods of time for the patient to talk with you, rather than one long period. This lessens fatigue, and provides consistent attention which increases his feelings of security.

Allow the patient to express his feelings regarding the illness. Let him talk about what it means to him in terms of his daily activities, his occupation, his family life. Patients may attribute weakness to a degenerating heart, when in fact it may be caused by prolonged immobilization. Patient teaching and the initiation of activity in a carefully monitored progressive exercise program is important in preventing him from becoming a cardiac cripple. Often you will find the patient has a distorted view of his limitations which you can clarify. For instance, when the patient says, "This is the end of my sex life," the nurse might reply, "After recovery, most patients' sex life returns to what it was in the past." It is also important to acknowledge the patient's expressed feelings. "It's understandable that you are depressed now, but as you begin to get better, you will feel less nervous about your physical condition and have more self-confidence." "You will be less perplexed about your limitations as you convalesce, because we will keep repeating all the things you need to know." This last remark also tells the patient you expect him to recover.

Some patients avoid resumption of sexual activity, fearing it will cause another heart attack, or because their depression lessens desire. The health worker who takes a sexual history has a good indication of the patient's sexual involvement before illness. The spouse or sexual partner should be involved in the discussion so that an individualized plan can be made. Consideration should be given to any limitations imposed by the heart disease, such as pain or dyspnea caused by activity. Couple counseling, with emphasis on loving, pleasurable activity that may not culminate in sexual intercourse is helpful in reducing performance anxiety. Patients should be cautioned to avoid sex with new partners or sexual experimentation on the basis that it might arouse too much anxiety. Feeling comfortable with the environment and with one's partner eliminates unnecessary anxiety and restores confidence.

Assure the patient that he is watched and observed at all times. He may ask, "Will I die if I go to sleep?" The nurse can reply, "There is no indication that your condition will change any more while you are asleep than when you are awake. In fact, you will expend less energy asleep than awake." Since many patients fear that they may die while sleeping, assure him that he will be carefully watched even when asleep.

Talk to the patient about plans for his transfer to a general care unit. Mention the positive aspects of the move. "You have been improving every day and now you are well enough to leave the coronary care unit." Although the patient wants to leave, he may be fearful that he will not receive equally good care after the move. The nurse should comment on the good quality of the care he will get, since the personnel are specially trained in giving cardiac care. Never convey the idea that only the nurse in the coronary care unit can be helpful and knowledgeable, since it is not valid. Remember that such an idea will upset and worry the patient. He may even overreact to the situation and build up enough anxiety to endanger his cardiac status, and to land him back in the coronary care unit.

One patient expressed concern about his transfer from the coronary care unit because he was afraid he would catch some disease from another patient in that unit. He was told, "Although another person in that unit may look very sick, his illness lies within himself just as yours does, and cannot be given to anyone else."

Use other resources to help the patient work through conflicts that existed before his myocardial infarction. Because of his vulnerable state, these conflicts may have increased. For example, the patient may have become rigid and controlling. He refuses to have others tell him what to do. He is angry about his helpless state and the enforced restrictions. Let him know that these restrictions are temporary. The need for control may well be a pressure area that will influence his recovery and/or future well-being. Suggest that "Sometimes when people are under a great deal of pressure, it affects their physical health. It helps to know how to deal with these pressures. We have a member on our team who is an expert at talking with people about just that. How would you feel about talking with him?" Deciding whether he wants to be helped gives the patient a sense of autonomy while letting him know that you are concerned about his feelings. Encourage him to know himself so that he can learn what triggers his emotional upsets. Help him find alternative means of solving his difficulties. Don't put a psychiatric label on the patient, because he gets upset. He has enough problems already.

Before being discharged from the hospital, the patient should be encouraged to think about times and episodes in which he felt stress. By recognizing his pressure limitations, he can learn to control them. The use of techniques such as biofeedback, exercise, psychotherapy, relaxation techniques, or medication may be helpful in offsetting tension.

Discussion regarding control of diabetes, blood cholesterol and triglyceride levels, obesity, hypertension, and elimination of cigarette smoking should be included in predischarge planning. If the implantation of an artificial pacemaker (or coronary surgery) is necessary, the staff may need to provide education, support, and reassurance so that the patient will accept the procedure.

Be aware of how you present yourself to the patient. A calm, comfortable but concerned approach is best. Be aware of your tone of voice, facial expression, amount of direct eye contact, and degree with which you gesture. Speak simply and clearly. Don't use terminology that the patient can't comprehend, since this often alarms him. Divide the time you spend with the patient. Short but frequent visits are best. This helps the patient feel that he is being followed carefully and lessens his need to use somatic complaints as a bid for attention.

Be a good listener. Let the patient know you value what he has to say. Be alert to comments that reveal his anxiety or hesitancy in talking to you. If the patient states, "There were so many things I never got to do," or "I've heard that few people survive these things," you can say, "You sound worried, which is certainly understandable. You will gain confidence as time passes and your strength returns."

Provide as restful and pleasant an environment as the unit permits. Clocks and calendars help keep the patient oriented as to the time and date, especially in intensive care units where lights are on twenty-four hours a day.

As the patient progresses toward full recovery, provide an opportunity for him to attend group sessions for coronary patients. These sessions validate the worth of giving up smoking, sticking to restricted dietary regimens, learning to relax, and working at a slower pace. They also have a beneficial effect by providing a chance for the patient to express feelings and attitudes about his condition.

When a patient is out of imminent danger, he may feel so confident that he denies the presence of illness. This serves to protect him from the implication of what a coronary means in terms of the length and quality of his future life. At the same time, it prevents him from cooperating and participating in a therapeutic life-saving program based on prevention and rehabilitation. Group meetings enable him to become more realistic in assessing his reaction to his physical state.

The Patient Undergoing Renal Dialysis or Transplant

Properly functioning kidney tissue is necessary for life. Inadequate function results in the accumulation of waste products in the blood stream and alteration of the body's chemical balance. This results in a condition called uremia. When uremia is severe and life-threatening, dialysis is generally instituted. Dialysis involves pumping the patient's arterial blood through a coiled tube of thin cellophane-like material. This coiled tube is immersed in a bath of fluid which closely resembles normal blood plasma. Excess waste products that have accumulated in the patient's blood are washed out through the coil membrane into the surrounding bath, resulting in more normal blood plasma. The dialyzed (washed) blood flows from the coil into tubing that leads back to the patient's venous circulation. Some patients are dialyzed on a short-term basis for acute kidney failure such as may occur in poisonings, shock, burns, severe acute nephritis, or severe injuries.

Other patients require long-term dialysis for chronic renal failure when the course and prognosis are uncertain or in preparation or expectation of receiving a renal transplant. A patient on chronic renal dialysis usually has a permanent arteriovenous shunt implanted in an arm or leg to provide ready access to an artery and a vein, both of which are used in the dialyzing procedure. Since the shunts are often external, they may become uncoupled, accidentally or willfully. The patient will then bleed profusely, and may die if the tube is not clamped in time.

More recently, surgical preparation of the patient for chronic dialysis has leaned toward creating a permanent arteriovenous connection in the patient's arm or leg. Such an arteriovenous fistula has the advantage of being unexposed, i.e., it is totally beneath the skin. But, after it has been created an appreciable period of time must elapse before it is ready for use. There is also the disadvantage of an increased circulatory and cardiac burden.

The patient in renal failure may have subtle or acute signs that are of psychological significance. However, it is important to realize that the symptoms are probably not related to the patient's emotional stability. Instead, they are related to the presence of toxic products in the blood stream which affect both brain and general nervous system functioning. Often a health worker may mistake the patient's symptoms (rambling, impaired ability to concentrate, complaints of headache, poor attention span, sleepiness, lethargy, twitching and/or confused state) as being the onset of an acute psychotic episode. In fact, they are the signs of an existing medical emergency. The symptoms disappear as treatment for the kidney failure is initiated and maintained.

Patients undergoing dialysis have a chronic medical condition. Many stresses are encountered by the patient as he adjusts to the treatment program. As happens with other patients who are subject to long-term, unending care, the physical limitations, as well as economic and social adjustments, create problems that have a psychological effect on the patient. It is helpful for the nurse to understand that the patient's behavior is a reaction to these pressures.

The patient's personality before illness and his coping skills when under stress are an important factor in his adjustment to dialysis. Patients who are able to tolerate frustration and can be optimistic regarding their situation appear more cooperative with the demands imposed by their illness.

The chronic dialysis patient looks forward to a confining life during which he is dependent upon a machine to which he is attached for almost an entire day or night two or three times a week. This dependency can be resented and feared. It can also create a great deal of anxiety, as it seriously interferes with the individual's ability to perform the work and/or household duties that he effectively managed before. The fear of losing his job and its income, and no prospect of complete recovery, often lead to a severe depression. A patient's tearfulness, lack of desire to talk, and disinterest in what is going on about him, is related to this depression, as are his loss of confidence and self-esteem.

Socially, the dialysis patient may not be able to keep up with the pace he previously enjoyed. Friends and family may begin to regard him as totally unable to function, helpless, and ill. Hence, they may unwittingly begin to relate to the patient as if he were incapable of thinking or answering for himself. The loss of self-value often comes about as a result of the patient's regarding himself in the same way that he thinks others regard him. If the patient begins to feel that those around him feel he is worthless, he may begin to believe that it is so. A man may no longer be called upon to act as the head of the household, or a woman may no longer be regarded as a competent mother and wife. An adolescent may be avoided by friends and rejected by school clubs because she cannot share in many extracurricular activities. In addition, the physical changes, especially the inability to urinate normally, causes considerable difficulty during adolescence, when the youngster is in the midst of developing a new body image. The sadness and unhappiness manifested in such instances may be so severe that the person may become deeply depressed and feel that death is really preferable to the life he is presently living.

The risk of suicide among such patients is high. The patient can kill himself easily by separating his shunt, which will allow him to bleed to death. Other suicide methods include refusing his dialysis treatment, or ignoring the dietary regimen (usually low protein, high carbohydrate and fat, low sodium and potassium).

Often the patient's emotional difficulty reflects itself in his inability to relate to the hospital staff. He may be a real problem in daily management and be unable to cope with even the simplest daily activities. His need for reassurance may take the form of a demand for constant attention from the staff. Irksome behavior may involve sounding the buzzer frequently and complaining almost continuously about seemingly trivial matters, such as the sheets not being straight or a chair being placed incorrectly. This behavior can become irritating to the staff, particularly if they do not understand that the patient is really saying, in the only way he can at that time, "Don't leave me; I'm afraid; I'm afraid to live; I'm afraid to die."

Some dialysis patients complain of intense nausea. One lady was so nauseated she could not retain any food whatsoever. The staff did not believe that the patient was as nauseated as she complained of being and thought that she was being purposely unpleasant. Their anger and rejection of her created difficulty for the patient. Actually, the patient was nauseated because of her uremic state, but her anxiety and fear increased the already unpleasant symptom. As she eventually became more hopeful, she experienced less nausea.

Dialysis patients are worriers. Why shouldn't they be? They have a lot to worry about. And their worries, furthermore, are not imaginary. They are only too real, because the hardships and the discomforts are real. Patients worry about day-to-day living, a major concern being whether they will be accepted into a long-term treatment program. They wonder if they will ever recover sufficiently to enjoy a trip, a play, a shopping spree, or even if they will ever leave the hospital alive. One lady had a sister who died from kidney disease at the age of twenty-two, and she naturally questioned her own chances of survival. Patients worry that their spouses will desert them, or that the shunt will be repugnant to others who may view it. They fear that they will run out of money and become impoverished, and that they will be hated for being unable to help with the family plans and routines because of illness, thereby disrupting those plans. One young girl worried constantly about completing high school, having friends, and the possibility of dating, marriage, and pregnancy.

Frequently, patients will appear to deny their situation or illness. Denial often alarms the staff because they feel that the patient who doesn't talk openly and continuously about his problem is surely headed for disaster. This is not necessarily so. Often the patient talks about the weather, shopping, going home, lipstick brands, or baseball averages in an attempt to reduce anxiety and the overwhelming unpleasant and uncomfortable thoughts about what is happening. Thus, the individual protects himself, and focuses on something that is real to him in order to hang on to his rapidly decreasing sense of self-control. However, when the patient acts as if he is hearing for the first time what you have told him two hundred times, flagrantly eats the wrong foods, and participates in sports which increase the chances of a shunt separation, his denial must be regarded as a problem.

The patient who needs a transplant is aware that his condition is grave and can be fatal. He knows the misery of being in kidney failure, is fearful of dying, and sees the transplant as the only real hope for prolonging his life. Additionally, the patient sees a chance for a new life without his semipermanent attachment to the dialysis machine. He is grateful if a donor is found but, by the same token, he feels guilty and responsible for the possible shortening of the donor's life. Many patients, fearful of a negative response, avoid approaching relatives who are possible donors. At the same time, relatives may avoid the patient if they suspect that they may be asked to be a donor; they may feel guilty if they refuse, yet think that because the donation is only palliative, not curative, it is not worth the risk to themselves.

Potential kidney recipients go through many moods, varying from grief to happiness, as they wait for the news that an acceptable kidney donor has been found. One young patient, on hearing that her father's kidney was not acceptable for transplant, became deeply depressed. She felt that God had forsaken her and that she must be an especially bad girl for him to punish her so terribly. She felt she had been refused a new life and was unloved by her father (God). For a while she refused to talk or look at her father, and accused him of being her enemy. Another patient, who had been told that his sister's kidney was acceptable, was able to lessen his feelings of guilt about the donation by reasoning that his sister was comparatively healthy and that girls don't have to work because they marry and stay home. Thus he felt that one kidney was really sufficient for her.

After transplant surgery, there is always the risk of tissue rejection by the patient's body. Patients realize this, but fear of such rejection is tempered by the knowledge that some transplants last for lengthy periods. However, living with the thought that the possibility of rejection always exists produces a great deal of fear. Although the patient is no longer in need of dialysis, he often questions his own decision to accept a transplant, thinking that perhaps it would have been better to live attached to the machine than to worry so much about the possible failure of the transplanted kidney. Some patients have also expressed the fear of dying as a punishment for accepting someone else's kidney. The patient needs help in coping with the uncertainty as to whether or not he will live. He needs to talk about his personal feelings with a health worker who has come to terms with his own feelings about death.

Family members usually need a great deal of emotional support in handling the stresses created when a family member is undergoing dialysis or transplantation. They may feel useless or guilty if they are unable or unwilling to supply the needed kidney. They may also resent having to meet the many demands of the patient. The burden of personal care, transportation, dietary management, and finances is great, and can become wearing over a period of time. The quality of the relationships between family members and the patient may undergo subtle changes which may have detrimental effects on all concerned. This is particularly true if feelings of displeasure, resentment, anger, or disappointment are not brought out into the open and discussed. If disagreements and arguments occur, it is imperative for members to talk realistically about what bothers them, rather than bottle up their emotions because they are under the impression that such repression spares the patient. Feelings of antagonism are communicated subtly or otherwise, with the patient then feeling that he is unworthy of being included in family matters. He may also misconstrue family conversations, feeling that he is the subject under discussion, even though the actual subject may be as remote as the purchase of a new refrigerator.

Talking things over gives the patient the opportunity to discuss his feelings and reveal his concerns and attitudes, and allows for openness, honesty, and improved understanding between all.

If family members are overly protective and continuously try to please and do everything for the patient, they may encourage him to behave like a child. This can also increase the patient's guilt regarding the anger he feels, possibly leading to a severe depression. Finding a middle road is not easy. The family needs help in providing support while, at the same time, encouraging the patient to do whatever he can for himself. This will encourage the patient by demonstrating the family's belief in his capabilities. If the patient is on dialysis in the home, stress is increased due to disruption of normal family life and the increased medical responsibility undertaken by the family. The intelligence and closeness of the relationships between family members and the ability of all to adjust to change and tolerate frustration will have an effect on the degree of success of the treatment.

It is important for health workers to understand the usual emotional reactions of the patient on dialysis so that they can tolerate and cope with the stress. The patient often displaces his own anger onto the staff and may be unappreciative, or even resistant, to the medical regime. His attitude may lead to anger and punitive dictatorial attitudes on the part of the health workers. Occasionally, a staff member will react by becoming over-solicitous and overprotective in order to offset his own hostile feelings.

It is helpful to hold staff conferences in which particular problems are discussed and therapeutic approaches are planned. For example, the staff approach to the patient with many unrealistic complaints had been to convince him that life wasn't so bad. The staff changed their approach and agreed with the patient that his situation certainly was difficult, with many frustrations. They elicited suggestions from him regarding plans for his future. Not only did the patient decrease his complaints, but his self-esteem rose as his feelings were regarded and given special consideration by the health workers.

Recognize that some denial is essential for the patient to discount the overwhelming ramifications of his situation. However, recognize the difference between denial that is in the service of helping the patient live from day to day as opposed to that which is counter to his survival. For example, if the patient says he doesn't need his medication because he is well, he must be given factual information to encourage compliance.

THE APPROACH TO THE PATIENT UNDERGOING KIDNEY DIALYSIS OR TRANSPLANT

Allow time and opportunity for the patient to talk about his serious situation. Do not lie or try to minimize it, as the patient usually learns the truth through his sensitivity to the reactions of those around him. Never deceive the patient. When the patient tells you that he is planning to return to work soon, help him determine what actually can be realistically expected. Tell the patient, "You will be able to return to work eventually, if some adjustments can be made in the number of hours you work per day." Another approach could be, "It is quite possible that you might desire to look into a less strenuous line of work. Have you considered any other vocation?" Or "Many women have been able to earn an adequate salary by working from their homes. Maybe you and I can look into some of the opportunities available." Present an optimistic outlook.

Encourage and support hope. The patient needs to have positive thoughts about his future in order to cope with the adversity, ongoing dis-

comfort or pain, and concerns about prognosis. Positive attitudes of the
health workers can do much to carry patients through difficult times. Staff
should reinforce the idea that the patient is entitled to life, regardless of
guilt about past misdeeds and wrongs. Offsetting masochistic and depressive behavior patterns by supporting his right to life and by providing hope
will enable the patient to summon forth emotional strength needed to
face the future and its uncertainties.

Explore the patient's feelings toward having a shunt. Although he
may feel negatively about it, he will probably choose to have it when alternatives are presented and understood. Help the patient look at what he
can achieve even though there are limitations, rather than stress what he
cannot do. Always try to understand the patient's fear of death and dependency. Your interest and concern in the person may help boost his
deteriorating self-image.

Give unending support. Never abandon the patient. Even though it
takes time to institute dialysis treatment or to arrange long-term plans for
home dialysis, the nurse can still help by listening and stressing the hopeful
plans that are under way.

*Recognize that the patient's bizarre behavior may be due to symp-
toms of uremia.* At the same time, recognize the pressures that generate
unusual behavior. Help the patient to deal with that behavior, and at the
same time attempt to alleviate the underlying pressure and social problems.

Do not tell the patient that all the problems are imaginary. Do not
tell other staff members that the patient needs a psychiatrist because his
problems are all emotional. He has enough difficulties, and such an implication may serve to reduce his already dwindling self-esteem. Reinforce
any ego strength he may have. Tell the patient, "You are in a very rough
situation. It is understandable that you are depressed. We will do whatever
is necessary to help you through this uncomfortable period."

*Teach the patient what to do in case of an accidental shunt separa-
tion.* Answer all his questions fully and honestly.

Discuss the pros and cons of a transplant with the patient. Patients
have few possible alternatives. Therefore, the positive should be emphasized, along with a discussion of what can realistically be expected. Tell
the patient, "You can be well for years. Rejection is something that may
always have to be reckoned with. If it should occur, it will have to be
handled in the best way possible at that time." Emotional difficulties

following transplantation are the rule, not the exception. All patients have psychological reactions. Therefore, health workers should help prepare the patient for the usual and anticipated reactions.

Be alert for signals that indicate the possibility of suicide. Continue to work with the patient on new solutions to problems that may arise.

Support relatives and allow them to talk about their feelings. This may not alter the patient's condition or the situation, but it is helpful in obtaining temporary relief from intense pent-up feelings. Your warmth, calmness, and sense of hopefulness helps them to feel stronger as they bear their heavy burden. It also boosts family morale.

The Pediatric Patient

Patients of all ages have some difficulty in accepting and adjusting to a period of hospitalization. The child—because of his limited reasoning ability—has an even harder time. He cannot fully comprehend the reasons why he is in the hospital. He wonders why he must undergo procedures that are often painful and scary, and why people who are in no way related to him are handling and poking him when all he wants is to be with his parents.

The child can never be fully prepared for hospitalization. For him it simply means being away from his home and separated from his parents, grandparents, siblings, and friends. He may be there because of a condition of sudden onset that threatened his life, or he may be there for elective surgery. Often, the pediatric patient's stay in the hospital is fairly short, but some children with chronic or terminal illnesses will spend many weeks or months in the hospital. A child who is uncomfortable and in distress may accept hospitalization more easily than one who is unaware that he has a problem. If he has been in an accident and requires immediate treatment, it may be impossible to provide an adequate explanation. It then becomes important to spend time with the child afterwards, to review what has happened and why certain procedures were done.

Because children have limited experience with illness, and are less able than adults to handle frustration, anything that can be done ahead of time to prepare them for events to come is generally helpful. Simple, matter-of-fact explanations of what is going to occur, where, and who will be there, allay anxiety. In cases of elective admission, the child's fears and apprehensions can be lessened by giving him a tour of the pediatric unit, and letting him see the sleeping and playing accommodations and having him meet some of the patients. In the prehospital visit, the child should be made aware of the pleasant features of hospitalization, such as continuous parenting, toys, playroom, books, as well as the pertinent unpleasant features, such as medications, tests, and treatments. To reinforce understanding, some hospitals have prepared booklets which describe almost everything that a child will experience. Allowing the child to have a part in planning for his hospitalization helps him feel he has some control over what is happening. It is always better to be truthful about what is to happen than to have the child draw conclusions, which are usually far worse than the reality. When there has been no preadmission visit, it is important for the staff to display genuine interest in the new patient and spend time with him. When the child feels up to it, just telling him about the unit is better than nothing and may help dispel much fear regarding what might be behind certain curtains or doors.

A child's logic is not the same as an adult's. He has his fantasy world —his inner psychological world—to which he responds, and this may differ from what is actually happening as the adult sees it. For instance, a child cannot understand that it is helpful for him to be in the hospital and that what is being done to him is really necessary. He cannot foresee that regaining his health and being well is worth going through an unpleasant experience. Rather, he may feel that what you say is good for him is really terrible. He may very well feel that the hospital is a prison and that he has been put there because he was "bad." He may worry about being punished for snitching those dimes, eating the forbidden candy, pushing his little brother downstairs, wishing something bad would happen to his mother, or for having masturbated. A child can easily feel that he must certainly be the very worst person alive for all this to be happening to him. He is sure his parents are angry with him. Why else would they have left him here? He hears no familiar voices. His brothers and sisters cannot come to visit him. He can't go out to play, and no pets are allowed. Practically speaking, personnel on the unit cannot replace the continuous care and presence of family members. Is it any wonder that he feels resentful toward the doctor, the nurse, and others who, he rightfully feels, are keeping him where he doesn't want to be and who are doing some very unpleasant things to him?

Hospital policies have relaxed increasingly in recent years to permit continuous presence of parents. This is particularly important for a child who fears separation from his mother and wants the attention, emotional comfort, and security she can provide. Sometimes hospital routines are disrupted by the presence of family members on the unit. However, that is a small price to pay for the valuable physical and emotional care his family provides for the child.

A child's sense of trust is strongly influenced by what his relationships with adults have been in the past. If his parents have lied to him repeatedly, even though they felt they were protecting him at the time, he will be less likely to accept what others tell him. Previous hospitalizations and experiences with medical personnel will also influence his expectations. For instance, the smiling professional who pats the child complacently, says, "Everything is just fine," and then orders unpleasant restrictions and tests lays the foundation for suspicion during future encounters. The child, like the adult, fears what he does not know, has not seen, or does not understand. However, the child obviously knows less, has seen less, and understands less than adults. Thus, making the unknown known to him, and hence increasing the child's understanding, may have a beneficial and soothing effect. Pretending to give a doll a hypodermic or intravenous injection, being allowed to play with an oxygen mask, being asked to hold cotton, tape, applicators, or tubes of ointment, helping prepare one's special feeding, seeing pictures of other children in situations similar to his own all help to make the hospital experience more understandable and hence more bearable.

The child brings all of his fears with him to the hospital. These fears —real or imagined—may be due to previous experiences, or they may be based on bits of conversation overheard at home. For example, he may have heard his mother talk about a neighbor who went to the hospital and then died, and conclude that this, then, is what is in store for him. Perhaps his grandmother had a heart condition and died from it. The child may feel that this is the natural outcome for all those who have heart trouble. Or he may believe that his broken leg is a punishment for disobeying his parents who had told him not to climb trees. These partially comprehended situations instill very real fears in a child because he has not yet learned to reason logically. Thus, the child views the hospital environment as a dangerous and threatening place.

In addition to the stress of his physical illness, the child must cope with separation from his parents—a traumatic experience in itself. Children do not like to feel helpless. Being removed from persons on whom the child is necessarily dependent increases this feeling, particularly when he cannot accept what others are doing to him. He is not consulted about plans that are made for him. He feels at the mercy of others, confined, trapped. He responds by protesting in the only ways he understands—he cries, shoves, hits, kicks, and throws things. He may refuse to eat, become withdrawn, avoid looking at you or responding to your approach, and refuse the toy you offer him. He is angry, resentful, unhappy. He wants to see his parents, but when they come his happiness at seeing them gives way to his unhappiness and he may cry and cling to them or remain silent and ignore them. All too often, such behavior is interpreted by the staff as indication that "the poor child is so upset by his parents' visits that he would really be better off without them." On the contrary, crying and silence are both pleas for affection and support, for help and hope, as well as outlets for tension and anger.

Parents' reactions to their children stem from their own background. They see their child's behavior as a reflection of how poorly they have brought him up, and this makes them feel inadequate. Spontaneously, their anxiety level rises and they may berate, admonish, and threaten the child, which only makes him feel worse and increases his fear. The health worker who is not judgmental in such instances can do much to help parents change the situation by encouraging them to give the child extra attention and to demonstrate their affection for him.

Some children are so undemanding, accepting, and uncomplaining that they are seen as perfect, lovable little models of adults. Because they do not pose management problems, they tend to be overlooked by staff members who give most of their attention to the loudly protesting children. However, these children are the ones who often need more attention than those who are noisy and demanding. They may be extremely inhibited and unable to demonstrate any aggressive behavior. They may believe they are hospitalized as punishment and will be released only if they behave perfectly. Often they submit to everything without a murmur out of fear of what will happen to them if they do not.

Reactions to separation vary in light of each child's previous experiences with his parents. It is not uncommon for a child to engage in regressive behavior—including bed wetting, refusing to eat, and using "baby talk"—as reactions to the stress. Health workers should understand and accept such regressive behavior for what it really is.

Children have limited ability to cope with frustration. During their early years, they demand immediate satisfaction and seek pleasure naturally and instinctively. Since the child's ego is not yet developed, he cannot deal with the adaptations required of him in this new and uncomfortable environment, and his reactions may seem irrational and emotional to adults. The healthier the child's development has been, the more secure he is, and the more consistency he has experienced, the better able he will be to deal with his present frustration. However, he may manifest his inability to deal with it by having a tantrum, hitting his head, sucking his thumb, throwing up food, and assaulting others. At such times, the worker allows the child to release his tension but protects him and others from injury. An attempt to help the child face the situation by acknowledging his predicament, rather than offering excuses, is helpful. The staff can share his feeling and show him that he is accepted by providing substitutes for the family love he is missing. This can be done by holding, cuddling, talking, and participating in an activity with him. At the same time, the health worker must begin to introduce the child to healthier ways of satisfying his wishes and obtaining attention. Often, putting the child with peers who exhibit more acceptable types of behavior, and pointing out how other children are able to obtain satisfaction, will induce him to perform in a like manner in order to gain peer acceptance.

All children fear being unloved, uncared for, or abandoned. Any separation or illness increases this fear. The health worker must understand that being hospitalized for any length of time is almost impossible for the child to endure and, because he does not yet have a sense of time, it seems to be lasting forever. A child does not understand the meaning of "Wait just a moment," "It will be over in a little while," or "I'll be there in a short time." Minutes seem like eternity. The notion of the future, soon, or later are too abstract for the young child. It is more helpful to respond to his questions by referring to the present.

Sometimes a child's reactions are based on unconscious conflicts, as when unhappiness is carried over from a previous experience. Fortunately, most children are quick to express their feelings. It is important to listen to them in order to pick up clues to hidden but real meanings in their reactions. Often what a child reacts to is not obvious to the adult, but bear in mind that all behavior has meaning and that the child's behavior is his best way of expressing himself. Thus do not fall into the trap of accusing a child of malingering or purposely "carrying on," or of being a "phony."

He is not, and what is more, he does not comprehend most of his own reasons for his behavior.

It is important for the health worker to take into consideration the relationship between the child and his parents and the parents' attitudes and demands which affect the child during his hospitalization. The worker will benefit if he can develop a good relationship with the parents by providing support, counsel, and information regarding institutional practices and the child's care.

Parents require help in dealing with their own reactions to the child's illness. If a child is fatally ill parents will react with shock, disbelief, and denial. Advances in treatment of incurable illness often extend the period of dying, but necessitate frequent, repeated hospitalizations. This causes much anxiety and anguish for the grieving family. It is not unusual to find family members displacing their anger about their tragedy onto the health professionals, God, or each other. Health professionals must be careful not to personalize the parents' criticism, but to meet it with understanding and support and to accept their difficult behavior as a symptom of distress in a trying situation.

A child's chronic illness is often too painful a burden for friends or others outside the family to share. Family members are often avoided by outsiders, who seek to protect themselves from the thought that this could also happen to them. As a result, the expression of grief is limited to the family unit. The health worker is often the only outside person strong enough to allow the family the opportunity to vent their feelings.

Children do remember what happens to them. Too often the hospital experience is embedded in the mind so deeply that it becomes the basis for a life-long emotional problem. The health worker should make every effort to alleviate pain and decrease frustration. Only people who genuinely enjoy being with, caring for, and communicating with children, should work on these units. Staff members should also be able to work with the parents, who may become overprotective when a child's illness is chronic. This can result in preventing the child from enjoying and developing his ability to the fullest that his life will allow.

A child's reaction to any loss that he suffers results in a variety of responses which offer clues as to the depth of his feelings. The precipitating event may be the loss of a body part, lack of availability of his parents, or separation from his siblings and playmates. His responses may fluctuate from a sad mood to irritability, or he may provoke others by hostile actions, voice numerous complaints of aches and pains, or chastise himself for being "bad." One child with severe burns was overheard frequently sobbing and repeating, "I'm a bad boy." He had been burned during an apartment house fire and believed this must have been a punishment for misbehaving in school.

The nurse should learn as much as possible about the child from his parents, especially facts about his feeding and toilet habits, since they carry so much significance. She may have to set aside some of the hospital rules and provide a less disciplined atmosphere in order to lessen the child's anxiety and increase his feeling of security. A child may fear punishment if he does not eat, humiliation if he wets the bed. The stress of separation often causes regression to an earlier type of problem and may induce enough anxiety to cause bedwetting. The nurse should assure the child that he will not be punished or rejected for this regression. By avoiding attitudes that reinforce fear and anxiety, and by expressing warmth and tenderness, the nurse can help to reduce the child's feeling of self-devaluation. Such attitudes can also help to reduce a child's fear of retribution based on previous experience in his home—an important point, since the anxiety such fear causes can adversely affect the outcome of the illness.

An explanation by the nurse of procedures that will be carried out will help to reduce the parents' own anxiety. It will also help them prepare the child for whatever is to come, and deal with his reactions to it. Keeping them as informed as possible, anticipating some of their concerns, and providing adequate explanations for what is worrying them can be very helpful to the child's parents.

THE APPROACH TO THE PEDIATRIC PATIENT

Establish a friendly relationship with the child. Talk with him, especially when his parents are not present. Speak to him as you would to a friend, respecting his unique feelings, desires, and needs. Do not use "baby talk" or speak as if he doesn't matter. Be aware of what you say to others when within his hearing. Go along with his way of doing things providing it does not interfere with his therapy. Do not be critical. Accept the child for himself and show an interest in his interests.

Help the child deal with problems as they arise. Keep him informed, in simple terms, of what is taking place. Be truthful. Recognize the fears and fantasies that he may have. Offer honest explanations and genuine reassurances that offset inaccurate beliefs.

Do not approach a child patient when you are overly anxious about something. He will pick up additional insecurity from you.

Do not overwhelm the child with facts and explanations. Instead, encourage communication using whatever materials (drawings, pictures, equipment) necessary to help him understand what is happening. Answer questions as they are asked, on a level that he will understand. Children fear pain and worry about harm to their bodies. Give reassuring, brief explanations regarding what is happening. Remember that avoiding the subject does not lessen anxieties, but leads to fantasies that are usually much more frightening than reality.

Recognize that the child sees any limitation (food, fluids, activity) as punishment. Being examined may also be viewed by a child as a form of punishment—a way of checking up on him. Remember that the child will not thank you for your wonderful care. Tolerate his behavior when he pushes you away and says, "I hate you," but continue to approach him and show genuine concern.

Understand how difficult it is for a child to wait. Try to take care of his physical needs as quickly as you can.

Provide outlets for the child's hostile feelings. Let him hit a doll, pound clay, cut paper, or draw pictures depicting his experience. Allow adequate play time. Provide dolls, doll house, table, chairs, unbreakables, push-and-pull toys, drawing paper, watercolors, crayons. Encourage drawing, since free drawing may disclose his inner feelings.

Arrange for a story-telling time. Do not use stories that depict horror, hurt, sorrow. Encourage the child to make up stories because they may give the worker insight into the child's fears or a difficult family situation.

Give a child a choice only when you know you can respect his decisions. Do not ask him if he wants a treatment when you know he will be made to have it even if he says no. Let him help with procedures when possible.

Encourage the parents to ask questions, and answer them truthfully no matter how upsetting the facts may be. This does not preclude helping to alleviate their feelings of guilt by explaining: "It is well known that the best precautions in the world cannot prevent this condition." "Children break legs and have other accidents, whether parents are there or not." "A child's curiosity and zest for pleasure is primary; therefore, he doesn't think about the dangers involved in what he wants to do."

Do not assume that because of your greater knowledge of behavior that you are better for the child than his own parents. If you do, you are meeting your own needs to be a mother or father. If a child of your own is hospitalized, assume the role of parent, not health worker.

Come to terms with your feelings toward your own parents. If you don't, you may react to the child's parents as you would to your own.

Health workers should be aware of their own feelings and reactions to the child whose condition does not improve. Often a very sick child is avoided just when he needs the staff's presence. Instead of deserting the child, all the resources that are available in the hospital should be brought in. This includes social workers, psychologists, and various special therapists. If the child's physical condition permits, close cooperation should be maintained with the school to help the child maintain his grade school level.

Be flexible. Be prepared to change plans as the child's condition changes rapidly. Daily plans are best, and provide the most satisfaction, especially when a child has a long-term illness. Flexibility is particularly essential when working with children. Give the child advance warning of when he will be needed for any tests or procedures, so that he can end his activities beforehand.

The Adolescent Patient

The adolescent is a vacillating combination of dependent child and independent adult. Even as he yearns for freedom to make his own decisions, he clings to the security of parental authority. He fights for autonomy and adult responsibility, yet is grateful for limitations that protect him from situations for which he is not ready.

The "growing up" years are often referred to as the best years of one's life. This may be true for some, but for most people it is true only in retrospect. In reality it is a turbulent period of doubt, insecurity, mixed feelings, and struggles, all intermingled with joys and sorrows. A glance at the years from ages thirteen through nineteen will show how tremendous are the emotional, social, and behavioral changes demanded of the adolescent. This period may present severe problems, depending on the particular healthiness or unhealthiness of the individual and his family.

The adolescent may frequently find himself unable to satisfy the overwhelming and divergent demands of self, family, school, and peer group. At these times of crisis, he needs to relate to individuals he feels he can trust, so that he can discuss, dissect, understand, and resolve new as well as daily problems that arise. Prevention or early intervention in adolescent difficulties is needed, regardless of whether the problems are of organic or purely emotional origin.

Adolescents are prone to intense feelings of love in which another person becomes the object of adulation. Usually the love object is someone who is secretly admired, older, and possesses wisdom, a special skill, or provides a unique service. It is not unusual for the health worker to become a love object while the patient is in the hospital. The youngster usually fantasizes about various aspects of the relationship, embellishing it far beyond the real situation. Often the adolescent interprets a kind comment or action by the love object as an intense sexual interest.

The adolescent may not talk about his feelings to the individual, but may act them out by making special requests, writing affectionate notes, or talking to a peer about his secret desires. He may even allude to a planned time for physical intimacy with the idolized person. The adolescent's strivings are an unconscious attempt to feel loved and needed by an important and idealized individual, who may be a teacher, movie star, health worker, or sports hero. Health workers who find themselves the object of such feelings should recognize the meaning and importance to the youngster and accept the flattery and affection in a sincere, genuine manner. This reassures the patient that his feelings are being taken seriously. At the same time, the reality of the relationship must be gently presented, in a manner that reaffirms his status as an appealing, intelligent person.

Every encouragement should be given to the development of appropriate relationships by the patient with others, through providing frequent visiting periods with those (particularly peers) who can supply his unmet needs for friendship and a mutually reciprocal relationship.

Until recently, the adolescent problem years were, for the most part, ignored or glossed over. Parents and others expected that they would be lived through, with all their funny, awkward, and, from the adult view, minor dilemmas. Yet some of the problems of this age group seem earthshattering to the adolescent. He may be going through an identity crisis, not knowing who he is or what he wants to be. Social events may be marred by a face full of pimples; gym may be consistently missed because of painful menstruation. Adults compare these problems with their own— making a decent living wage, for example, or keeping the house in order. By comparison, adolescents may seem trouble-free. The adult is often so busy with his own pursuits and problems that he doesn't have time or patience to listen, nor does he seem to understand when he does listen.

Today we know that time does not always erase the awful effects of mishandling of youngsters who have difficulties but receive little help during adolescence. They feel lost if they are not treated with dignity and

respect or if they receive little compassionate understanding and are seemingly misunderstood, discredited, and judged critically on the basis of
appearance and behavior only. If we are to intervene, we must begin to
comprehend the adolescent's viewpoint. How does he feel about the world
he lives in? What pressures does he feel, and what conflicts does he face?
We must recognize that the child brings to adolescence all of his childhood
insecurities, anxieties, and needs. Similarly, his previous conditioning will
manifest itself in his reaction to struggles and problems that arise when he
is subjected to the stresses of illness. This is particularly true when his
freedom is restricted, when he is completely immobilized, or when he has
to cope with hospital authority figures. It is therefore important for health
workers to apply what is known about adolescents when dealing with
them both in the community and in the hospital.

The adolescent's concerns about his schoolwork, career goals, involvement in drug use or sexual activity needs to be recognized, with
guidance and counseling made available. An appreciation of the special
needs of these youngsters by health workers is a basic factor in establishing
a therapeutic relationship. For example, a sense of deprivation may engulf
the adolescent as he is separated from friends, close family, and pets
during his hospital stay. Helping him deal with the impact of this temporary isolation is crucial. The health worker should encourage rational
thinking by pointing out the realities of his situation. For example, a lack
of visitors should not be interpreted as meaning that the whole world is
against him or that no one cares about him.

As adolescent girls experience changes in their physical appearance,
they often incur attention and teasing, particularly from boys. In the same
vein, boys are often teased about their high-pitched voices or their lack of
height. Boys may begin to have nocturnal emissions. Both sexes become
aware of new feelings and sensations and of the new interest of others. It is
as though the changing body has caused others to take note of a new and
meaningful person. Much emphasis is put on increased awareness of sexual
feelings and impulses. The adolescent is often in conflict between the wish
to fulfill his desires and the restrictions and prohibitions imposed by family or society. As his sexual drive and awareness is at a peak, he finds himself frustrated on the one hand and fighting for self-control on the other.

Adolescence involves a loss of old childhood friendships and a seeking of new relationships. New peer group loyalties become intense and are a mode of seeking support from friends, while loosening dependency ties to one's family. The peer group serves to diminish the feeling of being alone. Some adolescents involve themselves in romances. If this meaningful social relationship ends, the adolescent who is also alienated from his parents may feel that he actually has no one to whom he may turn and, in his loneliness, becomes very vulnerable.

The adolescent feels the need to establish a personal identity. In his search to find himself, he begins to be assertive. His quest for autonomy is often interpreted by the family as being a threat to them—a contradiction and condemnation of parental standards and demands, and a hostile reaction purposefully intended to hurt them. Instead, that need to find his identity is actually a maturational crisis, relevant to the adolescent phase of development. As a consequence, disruptions occur in what was once looked upon as a peaceful family existence. The adolescent sees his behavior as reasonable, justified, and meaningful. He sees himself as being able to make decisions concerning his own well-being, including the choice of foods, clothing, hair style, and friends. He may disassociate himself from his family and align himself with causes, groups, and even daring activities. In doing so, he often must deal with opposing parental reactions, which he views as interference with the establishment of his independence. Indeed, this assumption is often correct, because some parents threaten withdrawal of financial support, physical abuse, or deprivation of emotional support if their adolescent children do not comply with their demands. His parents' reactions have a deep effect on the adolescent's development of his autonomous self. The dilemma between the drive for independence and the still-present dependency gives rise to conflicts which generate much anxiety and uncertainty.

Conflicting attitudes between parents regarding each other's roles in the family will affect the adolescent, resulting in further confusion about his own identity. For instance, if the mother believes in permissiveness and the father is a rigid authoritarian, the mother may undermine an already difficult relationship between adolescent and father by creating situations in an underhanded way that enable the youngster to obtain more freedom behind his father's back. The message the adolescent then receives is that women must use subterfuge and dishonesty in order to have an ongoing relationship with men. If the adolescent is a boy, he may become suspicious of the motives of all women with whom he has relationships in the future. If the adolescent is a girl, she may adopt these same coping mechanisms for herself. All the while, the adolescent may feel that something is not quite right, and become increasingly uncertain of himself, as well as angry at his parents.

Parents are often stunned by the sudden changes in their child. They do not realize that a total lack of teen-aged rebellion could be a sign of regression. Normal adolescent behavior may include a derogatory attitude, unusual dress, foul language, and opposition to parental control of activities. These are ways of being an individual and asserting oneself. However, such behavior gives rise to much anxiety when parents do not trust their children to act without parental direction. Even those who claim they do often respond to their children's actions defensively. They see the adolescent's behavior as a blatant contradiction and "put-down" of themselves. They often unfairly interpret it as a war that has been declared, a competition between themselves and their offspring. Their anxiety is so heightened that they perceive only the negative characteristics of the behavior and ignore the positive ones. Parents ridicule, condemn, and tear down their youngsters in response to their own intrapsychic defensive operations. All of this adversely affects the youngster's development of his ego identity.

The family situation through childhood has an important bearing on adolescent behavior. When parents have always communicated with massive threats, the adolescent may respond by severely inhibiting his actions. This may result in so many restrictions on himself that dependency and a need for approval remain problems all his life. The adolescent in such a situation may displace his hostility from his parents to society in general. In families in which parents have been inconsistent, unconcerned, and have given little attention or discipline to their children, the adolescent may have difficulty in making decisions, have poor self-control, and find it difficult to accept any authority. Still another reaction may be found in youngsters who have been raised in an excessively strict home. Here the adolescent may rebel against any moral restrictions, and consequently develop conflicts caused by guilt feelings.

When parents shout, become upset frequently, and cannot control their anger, their child may react to his feelings in similar ways as he matures. That is, he may well displace his anger onto others. On the other hand, when the parents are generally fearful and resistant to change, they may discourage any free expression of self, or dissuade the adolescent from venturing into meaningful though difficult new undertakings. This may lead to a severe conflict in which the adolescent wants to be independent, but at the same time is fearful of assuming responsibility. Children who are overly protected and smothered with love are shielded from most responsibilities and prevented from participating in decision-making. As they become aware of their lack of experience in coping with ordinary daily problems, they become resentful, angry, and depressed. In a sense, they feel grossly short-changed. Their anxiety is so high that they are unable to function, often drop out of school, or fail to show up for work, and do very little but hang around the house.

However, not all adolescents have as difficult a time as we have described. Youngsters who are exposed to warmth and openness in their homes, whose achievements are met with approval and affection, and who are encouraged to be independent move forward into adolescence with a minimum of anxiety, concern, and dread of the responsibilities of adulthood.

The adolescent may affirm or condemn the life represented by his parents. He picks up the subtleties of parental conflicts, ambivalence, and fear of failure. He rebels against being used to satisfy the unmet needs of his elders, the vicarious living through him by his parents. For example, Sally observes that her mother spends lots of money at the country club, on clothes, jewelry, and at the beauty parlor. Sally's mother says that education is important, and regrets that she never had the opportunities open to Sally. At the same time, the mother frequently mentions the costliness of Sally's education, accuses her of not understanding the value of money, and demands that she demonstrate her appreciation of the sacrifices being made for her. Yet, when Sally is home on vacation and wears old jeans, Mother ridicules her appearance and remains aloof. Sally feels that she is being thrifty by wearing old clothes, and wonders why her mother doesn't love her for herself, instead of looking at materialistic articles. She persists in being herself. Mother goes into a rage because of her own need to conform and impress others. Her insecurity is partially due to her concern about other people's reactions to her. Her perception of the situation, however, is that Sally's behavior is hostile, and this leaves her frustrated. She threatens punishment. As a result, Sally feels misunderstood and withdraws in self-defense. She won't talk to Mother any more. At the time of her life that she most needs her mother, she becomes alienated from her. Sally feels that her mother's way of life is a hoax and lacks meaning. She is indignant because of the unfairness of standards preached but not practiced by her parents.

Parents may not have taken the time to know and understand their children because they have been preoccupied with their own interests, conflicts, and difficulties. Therefore, they will not know how to cope with the adolescent. They find it difficult to understand the meaning of new behavior patterns and almost impossible to accept the growth of their children's emotional independence and sexual and emotional investment in others.

During adolescence, one begins to think about possible occupations, the way one wants to earn a living, and the possible course of his life in regard to having a role in society. When jobs are scarce and the adolescent finds it impossible to find meaningful work, his sense of worth is lessened. He may feel that his driver's license and his social security card are society's only acknowledgment of his having grown up.

Many adolescents and their parents solve the lack of employment problem by using further education as a delaying tactic. Some teen-agers see college as an escape, or at least as an approved postponement of facing the adult world. In such a case, the student may find himself involved in intense scholastic competition which he cannot meet. He may be overwhelmed by all there is to learn, and unprepared for the lack of supervision or guidance in an environment less structured than that of his high school. Some find they are unable to develop their abilities or to meet parental standards. Others are bewildered, do not know what to study, and find the university gives them no direction in developing their talents. In large universities, students are often treated impersonally, and this may foster feelings of worthlessness. Dormitory life may also revive memories of infantile attachments to others of the same sex. Fears of intimate relationships when living closely together may throw an adolescent unsure of his identity into a homosexual panic. In short, college may really serve to intensify the adolescent's apprehensions and his feelings of inadequacy. All this may contribute to the current high suicide rate among college students.

The adolescent needs to reestablish trust and a sense of the worthwhileness of living in today's world. If his family is not available, it is up to the health worker to help him experience understanding, love, and dependability. The adolescent needs to feel autonomous and have a real sense of commitment. He needs to feel secure and guided by people he can trust, people who will not retaliate when he attempts to work through pressures and problems, whether they stem from his childhood, present encounters, or future uncertainties. He needs time and understanding to resolve tensions set up by personal change, distrust of adults, and environmental chaos. He welcomes limits that offer security by protecting him from his own undesirable behavior, while allowing him to attain a measure of adulthood.

The adolescent is struggling to develop his strengths. He may be enjoying or fearing the budding of his adult status and physical being. He is groping with adaptations in school, thoughts of a career, his changing relationships with others, his social obligations, and his home responsibilities. An illness can interrupt or even destroy his choices, possibly ending all hope for the realization of his plans and dreams. He needs support from the staff in determining what options are realistically available to him and what his limitations are. His family also needs direction in evaluating their hopes for him, as well as the pressures they are placing on him. Adolescence need not lead to constant turmoil of the youngster, family, and staff work together to assess and deal with the patient's valid needs.

THE APPROACH TO THE ADOLESCENT PATIENT

Understand the adolescent's need to mature. Whenever possible, include him in decisions that affect his care and treatment. Explain any procedures as completely as possible to alleviate his anxiety. Keep him informed about his progress during the treatment.

Do not impose your standards, beliefs, or values on him. Do not moralize. Rather, allow him to share his opinions, accept what he has to say, and agree or disagree without becoming defensive. Recognize the problems that exist without being judgmental.

Recognize that adolescent problems involve family interaction patterns. The patient's preadolescent relationship with his parents has set the stage for the present pattern. Do not threaten to withdraw your support in order to force him to live up to parental expectations. Instead, help him assess his position, as well as that taken by his parents; offer him encouragement without taking sides. Praise and encourage him when he makes independent decisions. Show that you care.

Treat the adolescent with dignity and respect. Do not belittle or discredit his ideas, friends, or romantic relationships. Regard his difficulties seriously. Do not call attention to his clothes, hair style, or choice of foods. Avoid speaking of academic achievement as the only worthwhile endeavor in life. Encourage physical activity to diminish tensions and anxiety. Stress the individual's positive characteristics. Do not look at normal adolescent behavior as though it were abnormal.

Set limits that are fair, and enforce them consistently. Recognize the special needs of the adolescent in order to prevent antisocial behavior while encouraging his growth of self-control. Help him channel his energies constructively through prescribed limitations.

Unless you genuinely like and care about adolescents, do not work with them if you can avoid it. Whether you do or don't like them, however, recognize your own fears, insecurities, anxieties, and drives, and do not displace them onto the adolescent patient.

The Patient
with a Postpartum Psychosis

Many people cling tenaciously to unrealistic notions of what marriage and parenthood are all about. They dream of romances between wholesome girls and boys who will love each other forever. Each will be aware of the other's needs, and be supportive. Finances and in-laws will never cause arguments, nor will any other problems arise. The wedding and honeymoon will be the beginning of an idyllic life together, which will be even more perfect after the arrival of each child. The bride and groom dream of matrimony and parenthood as devoid of difficulties. Love will conquer all!

If this has been one's expectation, consider the disappointment when the festivities of courtship and honeymoon are over and the realities of everyday living begin. With added responsibilities, psychological adaptations to a new mate, social pressures, and adjustments to their families of origin, both partners are apt to feel discouraged and disillusioned. Usually those who have sufficient ego strength and who have had a fairly healthy upbringing can weather the difficulties and work out a reasonable solution. They may make some compromises, but a new understanding of self and situation evolves.

The fact that most women learn to cope with marriage and motherhood may obscure the fact that it is not unusual for a woman *not* to be able to cope with the added stresses and strains which marriage, pregnancy, and motherhood impose. For such women, a pyramiding of various factors may result in a serious emotional problem following pregnancy. One should anticipate the possibility of postpartum illness in any woman who previously has not adapted well to extra pressures in life, who is having difficulty in her marital relationship, who experienced a serious trauma in early childhood, or who has a poor self-image. At times, pregnancy itself may activate an upset in one who has had a previous psychiatric illness. This is especially true if the person never fully resolved all her conflicts during the earlier period of treatment. In cases in which overt psychiatric problems were present before pregnancy, there may be a lessening of symptoms during the pregnancy. However, the original problems often reappear during the puerperium. Pregnancy may also activate repressed feelings about sex. Many women still have feelings of shame regarding intercourse. Pregnancy produces obvious evidence of a sexual relationship and may force these repressed sexual feelings into conscious awareness.

Emotional difficulties during pregnancy and following delivery are considered by some researchers to result primarily from physiologic changes in the body accompanying pregnancy, parturition (delivery), and the postpartum state. There is much evidence to support such a concept because it is known that changes do occur in thyroid, adrenal, and pituitary hormones during these times. On the other hand, it is also evident that postpartum emotional disturbances usually occur in those with a background of long-standing emotional problems.

A period of postpartum "blues" is fairly common within the first few weeks after delivery. In addition to the hormonal changes, there are subtle social changes for the new mother. Up to the time of delivery, *her* health status has been the center of focus. However, once the baby has been born, interest shifts to *his* welfare, *his* eating, sleeping, and defecation patterns. Some mothers are unable to cope with the shift of attention from themselves to this new person, to whom they often lack a sense of attachment. They frequently resent the intrusion of this demanding infant who does not recognize maternal needs for peace, quiet, and, above all, a good night's sleep. Once the attachment process begins, the "blues" usually disappear. However, the vulnerability to unconscious and conscious stresses are greater at this time, and symptoms of deeper emotional illness may appear, requiring immediate intervention.

Orientation programs for new jobs or new roles are standard practice in industry. Yet parenthood, a vitally important role, is often learned as on-the-job-training, without professional input. How much more therapeutic it is to use anticipatory guidance, including information and special help regarding the baby's care, and to give assistance in the adaptation to becoming a mother. Antepartum and postpartum classes are helpful for both parents as a way of providing support and as a vehicle for anticipating situations that may lead to physical or emotional difficulties.

In our Western culture, we tend to think that pregnancy, childbirth, and the bearing of a new baby are happy times for all. We sanction this ideal and give our approval to those who give "proper" responses. For example, we want to believe that every mother really wanted to be pregnant and that she is proud of her changing physical appearance. We also want to believe that the mother is really immersed in planning the infant's care, that she is fixing up the baby's room, taking child psychology courses, and shopping for the layette. If all this is so, we smile, pat her shoulder, talk about baby names, and even say that she will be a "good" mother. On the other hand, a woman who is unfortunate enough to feel otherwise has no eager or sympathetic listener. If she complains that she is not really ready to have a baby, or that she can't stand herself in maternity clothes, or that she doesn't know how to take care of a baby and fears doing so, she is turned off quickly. She may feel that she still needs mothering, that she still needs someone to take care of *her*. Even her smallest verbal indication that she is unhappy may provoke responses that let her know her remarks are unacceptable. "How could you feel that way?" "It's wrong to say what you're saying." "You'll see; you'll feel differently when the baby is born." "Don't complain. After all you got yourself into this. You have no one else to blame." These responses tell the woman she is not supposed to subscribe to her feelings, that she may incur punishment if she doesn't rid herself of them, that things will be better afterwards (although "after" may be what she fears the most), and that she is to blame for her predicament and thus deserves to suffer. Instead of the help she may be crying for, the woman who expresses her unhappy feelings finds that she has an additional problem. She now feels that she is "bad," thus increasing her guilt feelings about her thoughts, which are uncontrollable. Also, she may think that no one will be able to understand her feelings and, therefore, she tries to protect herself from any possibility of rejection, humiliation, and ostracism. Hence, even though she may want to seek help, she is afraid to do so.

The new mother encounters increased anxiety and fear about caring for the infant and all the implied responsibilities. If she is reticent or has misgivings regarding the baby's care, she may begin to feel that perhaps she doesn't love her infant as she thinks she should. The crying, frequent feedings, and diaper-changing are demands she may have difficulty in meeting. If the woman is not feeling physically and emotionally well, she usually cannot assess what is really bothering her. In the hospital, an alert nurse may observe that her sleeplessness, fatigue, and emotional lability are out of the ordinary, more than the usual postpartum "blues." The nurse may also observe that the patient is in an overly cheerful state, overly talkative, and that she engages in excess activity which accomplishes little. Most women experience a sense of unreality following delivery. It is difficult to believe that *this* baby was in the uterus. It is normal for the mother to be devoid of feelings of "motherliness," but she may misinterpret this as a sign that she will not be a "good" mother. She may be plagued by excessive fatigue as she wakens during the night to make certain that the newborn is all right. She may even have dreams of infanticide, with subsequent guilt feelings.

The new mother who is breast-feeding may have difficulty in getting the baby to suck. She may feel frustrated and angry, and fear that her milk is poisoning the infant, or that the infant will be smothered by her breast. The many chores, including having to be up at night for feedings, decrease the amount of sleep she gets and increase her feeling of being disorganized. At the same time, she may feel inadequate as a housekeeper if her standards are unreasonably high. She may be unable to keep her home in the same tidy condition as before the baby's birth and feel that she will never catch up with the housework.

If the woman has recently moved to a new location, she may begin to feel overwhelmed by everything and be unable to cope with her rising anxiety. In addition to having no one nearby for support, her family may be having financial difficulties. The woman may have given up a job with its second income, which had made her life easier. Now there is an added mouth to feed, and less money. If her husband's salary is not adequate, she may not be able to afford even temporary help, let alone a housekeeper.

Many women feel trapped in the home while taking care of small infants, and bored with the entire process. A woman who has held a fairly good job feels little status arising from her skills as a homemaker. Perhaps she went into marriage and pregnancy expecting sudden inner fulfillment, or anticipated that having a child would add new meaning to her life. Perhaps she wanted to prove to herself that she could produce a child, or that she was still young. She may have thought that the child would serve as a stabilizer for a rocky marriage—usually an erroneous idea. Instead of finding happiness in her new mother-role, she may become depressed to the point where professional intervention is necessary.

She may begin to feel hostile toward her mate in general, and the baby in particular, for causing all these problems. Hostile feelings may be intensified if the marital relationship was poor from the start. The husband may be insensitive and self-demanding, or he may just be the target for his wife's unhappiness. He may be blamed for the entire situation as her guilt regarding sexual relations increases and her feelings of inadequacy come into the open. Impulses, thoughts, and desires may focus on the wish that her husband would die and/or the possibility of killing the baby. These thoughts create so much anxiety that often the patient can not distinguish between what she did or did not do. Her thoughts and emotions are in conflict with what she believes should be appropriate for a new mother. She is considered psychiatrically ill if the problem becomes great enough to interfere with her ability to function effectively and satisfactorily for her own and her family's sake.

The course of the illness may assume one of two directions. In one, the mother may begin to feel more hostile and act on some of her pressing impulses and repressed urges. In the other, she feels she has failed as a mother, withdraws from the infant, and is overtly depressed. Whichever form the illness takes, the onset usually appears suddenly following the birth of the baby.

At times the patient may be in a completely uncontrollable manic state. She may swear and shout profanities. One patient raced through the psychiatric unit, taking off all her clothes, yelling, "I am a virgin, I am a virgin." Another continually sang, laughed, and cried to keep herself awake because she had a dream that the baby would die if she slept.

Again, depending on the course the illness takes, the patient may either lose all her sexual inhibitions or become completely uninterested in sex. Understandably, it is the relationship between sex and reproduction that makes sex so much a part of one's thoughts during the illness. Among

240 *Specific Approaches*

the sexual difficulties described by women are an inability to feel responsive or to reach orgasm. Often the woman has a difficult time admitting these sexual problems to herself or others, particularly if she wants to project a "femme fatale" image. Previous love affairs are remembered as failures because they did not culminate in marriage. Guilt, fear, and shame associated with intercourse are not uncommon, but usually are not confided to the spouse for fear he will laugh, ridicule, or accuse her of being half a woman. During the patient's illness, inhibitions are weakened, and a barrage of sexual ideas, words, and actions are apt to be heard. One patient started simulating intercourse, cursing the fantasized partner at the same time.

If the illness is of a depressive nature, sexual drive will be decreased or completely absent. Here the woman may feel guilt and shame about intercourse. She may fear another pregnancy, or perhaps she is too exhausted to participate in sex. A patient whose pregnancy terminates with the death of the infant may experience similar difficulties. In addition, she tends to blame herself for past misdeeds, seeing the death as a punishment for the real or fantasized behavior.

Emotional illnesses that develop following delivery are characterized by extreme fatigue and sleeplessness; extreme emotional lability with tearfulness at the slightest provocation; overconcern with minor aches and pains; expression of fears related to handling the baby; and inability to mobilize oneself. Delusions regarding oneself and others in the environment are not uncommon, and may include doubt regarding the husband's continued love, fear of his unfaithfulness, and the possibility of being deserted.

THE APPROACH TO THE PATIENT WITH A POSTPARTUM PSYCHOSIS

Listen to what the patient has to say. Offer a warm, concerned, understanding relationship. Avoid questioning the patient or probing for information with which to round out the history. She cannot discuss her experiences at this time; besides, uncovering them may lead to an increase in her disturbance. Avoid reminding the patient of what she has said that was either irrational or inappropriate. No doubt she has already forgotten what she said previously, and reminding her may cause a severe upset.

Give full attention when the patient talks about her symptoms. Do not slough them off as unimportant. Tell the patient that her symptoms can be relieved with treatment and medication. Emphasize the steps that have been taken in that direction—providing her with a quiet room, warm baths, activities to release tension, medication to help relieve discomfort, warm milk before sleep. Stress the availability of staff members.

Arrange for frequent and consistent one-to-one interactions. Two or three staff members should take turns with the patient during each tour of duty and provide continuous care while avoiding excess strain and fatigue of any one staff member.

Do not argue with the patient when she describes hallucinations or delusions. Tell her "You feel this way because of your illness. As you feel more comfortable and get needed rest, these thoughts will subside and be less bothersome." Help the patient to understand that her dreams did not really happen.

Do not appear shocked by ideas expressed in bizarre forms. Suggestive or seductive movements or remarks, or abusive and/or vulgar langauge are the result of a lowering of the patient's inhibitions, and the nurse should understand this.

Set reasonable limits. Help the patient to appreciate limitations and controls to avoid embarrassment to herself. Present reality to her. Deal with impulsive acts as necessary, e.g., if the patient starts taking off her clothes in the day room, say, "You are taking your clothes off in the middle of the day room. Now I will help you return to your room so you can dress." Then assist the patient to do so.

If the patient becomes uncooperative, obtain adequate help, and then take stern action. If she is unable to follow directions for her treatment and management, explain what you are going to do, the reasons why, and then act promptly. "You are being moved to Room 221 because it is quieter and the nursing station is closer, in case you should need someone."

Reassure the patient that her present feelings will be relieved as she improves. Tell her, "Some of these feelings are due to your illness." Don't give her cause to believe that she is not being a responsible and devoted mother. Accept her expression of her angry feelings toward her baby and husband but do not dwell on them. At this time she needs complete relief from thinking about the baby. Direct her into concrete and simple tasks, e.g., stamping envelopes, typing, clay modelling, recreational activities.

If the patient asks about her baby, answer truthfully. Present her with the reality of the situation in a kind, firm manner, saying, "Yes, you have a baby. He is fine and being cared for." If she is fearful of harming her baby, accept her fears calmly. Tell her that her baby will be well taken care of until she feels less anxious and can resume that care herself. If the doctor has imposed limited visits because of the patient's anger toward her infant and husband, tell her, "As your condition improves, the visits will be increased."

Inform the patient of any medication and treatment she will be given. Stress their benefit to her in terms of alleviating depression, reducing her anxiety level, allowing a good sleep, and bolstering her nutrition.

As the patient improves, discuss plans for her immediate future. Help her to plan for extra help when she goes home. Instruct her about how to secure financial assistance and how to use the services of the public health or visiting nurse.

If the patient's pregnancy ended with death of the infant, share her grief. (See approach for depression following loss, p. 75.)

The Aged Patient

What does it mean to grow old? Some of the meanings of aging can be discovered simply by taking time to become acquainted with the elderly. Not surprisingly, older people do not all feel the same way about aging. Those who enjoy their senior years see retirement as a time to pursue hobbies for which they had no time previously. They look forward to having fewer obligations, freedom to come and go as they please, time to sit and enjoy a good book.

Others feel that aging results in their no longer being needed. They see themselves as worthless because they are not earning a living. The decrease in their obligations is interpreted as an indication that no one wants them or cares about them. They have too much time on their hands, and do not know how to fill the many free hours that are available each day. Even when opportunities for activity are presented, they lack the energy and initiative to involve themselves.

The way one views his past life has much to do with the kind of person he is at, say, seventy. For instance, if a person feels he has had a comfortable life, with meaningful relationships, has accomplished some of his goals, and has achieved a sense of fulfillment within himself, he will tend to think of aging as a continuing, inevitable phase of life that has positive value. But if, in the past, the person viewed life as a hardship with many frustrations, and if his dreams and hopes have been unfulfilled, he will be likely to see his last phase of life as just another dead end.

By the same token, the aged person who has been active in his earlier years, has been a joiner, a doer, will usually continue to have an interest in

243

being with others and participating with them in various activities. He will continue to be involved in the life around him, even if he physically cannot do as much as he once did. One lady, who had been a professional nurse for forty years, became a much-needed hospital volunteer who read books and wrote letters for incapacitated war veterans. Physiologically, she could no longer carry the work load of the average nurse. But through her volunteer service she continued to be in touch with her profession in a way which gave personal meaning to her life.

The individual who always tended to remain by himself, had little to do with other people, had few personal interests save watching television and dozing in an easy chair, day in and day out, will most likely follow the same routine as he ages. Excluding those who develop senile arteriosclerosis, people's personalities do not change drastically as their faces wrinkle. The same positive and negative facets of the personality are apparent, or perhaps they become more accentuated under the stress of advancing years.

An elderly gentleman was admitted to the hospital with a history of a year-long depression which dated back to the day he had sold his gardening business because he was no longer able to do the physical work that it required. From early youth onward, he had loved nature and the out-of-doors. Virtually his entire life had been spent working by himself, caring for grass, flowers, and plants. He enjoyed seeing the results produced by his marvelously green thumb. His work kept him so involved that he never felt a need to bother with anyone or anything else. Retirement took away the one thing he had really depended on. Even his family was not aware of how little he had been involved with them throughout their lives. In fact, they could not understand his being so unhappy in a situation which they thought would bring relief from work and responsibility. When the nursing staff attempted to engage the patient in various group therapies, he barely responded. Fortunately, one nurse who had a great deal of insight into his problem arranged for him to take care of the plants on the unit. She also talked to his relatives and together they contacted a nursery that could, indeed, use the services of an elderly gentleman gardener. The pay was negligible but that was immaterial compared with the importance of finding a way in which the patient could pursue his lifelong life style.

The best way for the worker to find out how the aged patient sees himself and his past life, and how he feels about his future years, is to sit down and really listen to what he has to say. After all, he knows best what he really is all about, how he has managed all these years, what his habits have been, what works for him and what does not. For example, when an individual who is used to hot coffee and a pastry for breakfast, and has been enjoying it for sixty or so years, is suddenly faced with porridge, soft-boiled egg, and lukewarm coffee, he can be expected to lose his appetite completely. Any lectures by the young nurse on the subject of nutrition will be ignored or met with real anger.

Some staff members seem to have the attitude that older people have little need for privacy, few feelings, and no sexual ideas or urges. Patients tell us that the reverse is actually true. The older person enjoys a familiar, warm, well-lighted environment. He enjoys having a room of his own where he can keep his precious things and maintain a way of life that he can manage. He is sensitive, and needs attention to his individual needs. For instance, one elderly lady requested that her bed be placed near the window. The nurse refused, saying it was much too drafty there, and that the patient would catch cold. But it happened that the patient had lived most of her life in a cold climate and, contrary to most older people, never gave much thought to cool air or drafts. If she got chilly she would just put on a sweater or use an extra blanket. The stimulation and pleasure she would have derived from being able to see the happenings near the hospital entrance and parking lot would have given her an opportunity to feel as though she were participating in the life around her.

Sometimes staff members talk together in the presence of an older patient as if he were totally deaf. One nurse, while bathing a patient who was moving very slowly, turned and remarked to her coworker, "Boy, this one sure is a doozy. I'll never get my assignment done today."

When an older person desires or has an active sex life, he is often regarded as a "dirty old man." The staff on one unit actually requested a psychiatric consultation for an elderly gentleman who verbalized sexual feelings in relation to a young nurse. An elderly head nurse who sensed a "soft-pedaling" of conversation regarding sexual matters when she was present, remarked, "You know, some people may not believe this, but I had my day once upon a time. I was quite a live wire, went all over, had plenty of beaus and enjoyed them, too." The fact is that many older people continue to enjoy an active sexual life. A sexual relationship is often thwarted by practical problems that beset the aged. Where, when, and with whom are not simple decisions when one has experienced loss of spouse, friends, and relationships, and has housing, transportation, and financial difficulties.

Health problems of the aged can interfere with sexual functioning. Atrophy of the vaginal wall with a resultant decrease in lubrication, prostatectomy, diabetes, heart disease, stroke, severe arthritis, or emotional difficulties may play a large role in the geriatric patient's ability to perform sexually. Individuals who see themselves as physically repulsive, with bodies that are no longer firm, often avoid any physical intimacy. Men frequently worry that they will cease to have erections, and may therefore go overboard proving their potency and virility through increased sexual activity. They may seek erotic magazines or motion pictures in order to stimulate their waning desires. Insecurity regarding the individual's own sexuality may give rise to undue jealousy and suspiciousness, if the spouse relates to others.

Health workers who recognize that they are anxious at the idea that old people have sexual relations would do well to examine the origin of their feelings. One health worker, who was very angry when she discovered two elderly patients in bed together, stated, "I could never picture my folks having sex. Everyone else, yes. But not *my* folks. If I weren't here, I'd swear they never did it." In the discussion that followed, the worker was able to see on a conscious level that these patients bore a resemblance to her own parents, and that she had transferred her negative feelings about sex onto them. On an unconscious level, she was not aware that her negative feelings stemmed from her childhood and were a defense mechanism to control the discomfort she felt when sexually attracted to her father. The health worker's understanding of the origin of her attitudes helped her to be less judgmental about her own parents' sexual love. In addition, she became more tolerant concerning feelings of sexuality among the aged.

Frequently, staff members shy away from the aged person, because they find the changes that take place repugnant. Hesitant speech; occasional memory lapses; unsteady steps; wrinkled, dry skin; thinning, white hair; impaired hearing and sight; a tendency to react negatively to change; failing sensory and mental abilities are all reminders that a long life brings problems and imposes limitations. The nurse cannot turn the clock back thirty years and restore health and vitality to the aged patient, but she certainly can be aware of his needs, and incorporate them into her plan for his care.

Health workers may fall victim to the pressures of our culture which glorifies youth and seems to say that only the young are important. They may categorize all older people as fitting into a stereotype and be unable to see them as individuals. This attitude is reflected in the moans of a staff member who is told that her expected admission is a seventy-year-old lady. Before the patient has set foot on the unit, the nurse anticipates that her patient will be helpless, hopeless, and uninteresting—that she may need a great deal of extra attention, may make unnecessary noises, and be difficult and unrewarding to care for.

A pessimistic attitude on the part of the health worker is sometimes attributed to the idea that senility is rarely reversible. In many instances, it does progress as the individual continues to live. Even so, much can be offered to the aged in terms of therapy, including recreational therapy, occupational therapy, group therapy, and medications. Any or all of these may result in a lessening of distressing symptoms through improved contact with reality, increased motivation, and the reinforcement of appropriate behavior. Frequently, it is depression, rather than senility, which causes patients to behave in a nonfunctional fashion. Involvement of the patient often decreases the depression and allows the patient to take part in life again.

Projecting herself into the future may help the nurse to understand her elderly patients. Quickly, she will touch on not being active in nursing, her children grown and away, and her savings small (nurses were never known for their fortunes). Her friends and relatives may have passed on; her health may be failing. But while she is projecting this image, she will also do well to keep in mind that somehow she will be able to cope and survive. She will realize that she will want to make decisions about her dress, whom she wants to help her, and what she wants to do. She knows that she will not enjoy being ignored, treated in an offhand manner or as if she is "too old to know anything" because she has retired. Although she may expect to need a little assistance at times, she will not want to be treated as a child. She will expect that others will accept her as she is and not impose unnecessary restrictions simply because of her age.

THE APPROACH TO THE AGED PATIENT

Recognize that each person should be treated as an individual. Avoid categorizing older patients. Just because certain characteristics have been associated with the aged does not mean that all people have them. Give yourself the opportunity to know the person. Listen to what he has to say, what his life has meant, what his occupation and roles were, and what his present interests are.

Treat the person with respect. Realize that the "patient" role is not only difficult, but in most cases unsuitable and not beneficial to the personality. Tell him you will try to meet his needs within the limitations that the hospital imposes on you. Do not look upon his requests or complaints as silly, meaningless, or not worthwhile. Instead, explore troublesome issues with the patient.

When the patient becomes upset, withdrawn, or loses his appetite, try to understand what led to this behavior. Perhaps he can't remember who it was that visited him yesterday, or at what time his therapy is scheduled, or when meals are served. He may be unable to verbalize his frustration and anger at himself for not being totally competent anymore. He may begin to feel hopeless and either withdraw from everyone, or become irritable, antagonistic, or noisy.

Provide extra time in your daily schedule for the aged. They are not as agile as younger patients, feel more insecure, and want to be careful. Do not be critical when the patient is slow.

Understand your own feelings in regard to growing older. Consider how you think you would like to be treated when you, yourself, have grown old.

Don't talk down to the older patient. Oversolicitousness or overprotectiveness reduces his self-esteem and intensifies his feelings that you think little of him.

Be aware that patients respond to your verbal and nonverbal behavior. Actions sometimes convey more meaning than words. See that the extra blanket is available, the lamp is working, the coffee is hot, and the bedpan is removed soon after use.

Take physiological changes in the elderly into consideration. Speak loudly and distinctly, provide a night light to help prevent disorientation. Keep passageways clear of obstacles.

Do not use insincere phrases. "I know what it's like," "Things will be all right soon," or "You shouldn't feel this way; some people are worse off," are not only insincere remarks—they are also very irritating to the patient who recognizes them for what they are.

Try to interest the patient in activities. Occupational therapy activities, walking, cooking, or playing a musical instrument may appeal to the patient if the nurse arranges for them.

Provide close supervision for the potentially suicidal patient. Remember, even after a depression lifts, the patient will still need support.

Encourage the staff and the patient's family to convey to him the feeling that he is needed and wanted.

The Terminally Ill Patient

Perhaps no patient affects the emotional core of staff members more deeply than the patient with a terminal illness. The dying patient is in constant fear of losing his right to life, liberty, and happiness. The finality of the loss of one's identity, one's being as he has come to know it, is an overwhelming insult to the mind and body.

No one has a past experience with death. The experience belongs solely to the patient in the moment-to-moment happening. Regardless of the disease he may have, the terminal patient loses ground gradually, day by day, hour by hour. Sometimes he appears to improve markedly shortly before death, giving his family and friends hope that he will recover.

The patient may or may not have been told his diagnosis and may or may not know the truth about his condition. How much he knows depends on whether he expresses a desire to know. Often the family may make the decision to "protect" their loved one from knowing the truth. Many times the physician himself is not comfortable handling the subject. In one instance, the doctor could not bear revealing the unfavorable diagnosis to the patient or family while facing them. He used the telephone as his intermediary, and the effect on the person who received the call was devastating.

Regardless of what they are told, most terminally ill patients sense that something is not right. In fact, they know that things are drastically wrong. One such patient said, "I feel like I am in the midst of a personal disaster." The patient is aware that he is not getting better. He does not perceive slight improvements or gains. He recognizes, consciously or un-

251

consciously, that his life is coming to an end. He must cope, in some way, with what is happening to him. Most people have an awareness of their own mortality but dismiss thoughts of it as unimportant in the here and now. Essentially, if one dwelt on his anticipated death, he could not function in everyday life.

Dr. Kübler-Ross,[1] who has written much on the subject of death, has noted that the experience of dying progresses through several stages. At first, the patient *denies* what is happening and refuses to believe the diagnosis. He may seek other medical consultations, hoping that another physician will offer a more acceptable opinion. Once belief occurs, the patient may show great *anger.* Life is so cruel! He then tries to *bargain* for more time, usually making promises to his God in exchange for living to see some happy family event. *Depression* may then set in, as the patient realizes that his illness is in its terminal stages. (However, he has, in truth, been depressed even before this knowledge.) Finally, the patient is able to *accept* his fate, and finds peace within himself. He can then separate himself from everyone, and spends an increasing amount of time sleeping.

When a patient is informed of his prognosis, he may become so upset and bewildered that he is actually unable to hear and/or fully comprehend what he is being told. He may appear to be calm, and this may be interpreted as meaning that he has heard and understood. Later, he appears never to have been told for he heard only what he wanted to hear. The full meaning may be too shattering to accept, and the patient will ask the same questions over and over.

When a patient does not want to believe that he has heard the truth, he denies it. This mechanism is frequently encountered in terminal patients. It becomes apparent when the patient believes that he is improving and expects to get well rapidly. He may rationalize by telling others that he is being treated for a lesser condition, or that the doctors must be incompetent because they can't come up with adequate treatment for him or they haven't yet made up their minds as to what is wrong. Even when a patient admits verbally that he has a terminal illness, has apparently accepted it, and speaks openly about it, some denial is observed in his behavior. One patient stated, "I know I have a malignant cancer, but I am lucky that it was caught in time for a cure." This was not what the patient

1. E. Kübler-Ross. *On Death and Dying.* New York: The Macmillan Company, 1969.

had been told but what she had to believe. The coexistence of acceptance and denial is not unusual, and inconsistencies in the patient's verbalizations are most apparent to the staff.

The patient who is terminally ill with a painful disorder primarily worries about his level of comfort. He sees no end in sight to his constant pain. He fears the health worker will not bring his medication on time. As a result, he watches the clock, asking for his next dose earlier than allowed. His anxiety increases, making his pain even more unbearable. His entire day is spent concentrating on the probability that he will feel pain and that he will not get sufficient relief. It is much more helpful to administer the drugs in small amounts, on a regular basis, than to force the patient to wait additional time for one big dose of medication. Smaller, more frequent administration lessens the patient's fear that he won't get enough of the medication he needs. His certainty that his need for pain relief will be met encourages him to use his time and energy in other directions, making the quality of his life more acceptable.

This emphasis on preventing pain before or as soon as it starts, rather than treating it when it is severe, often forces health workers to examine and discard archaic attitudes regarding the addiction of terminally ill patients. The problem of potential addiction is more likely to result from providing too little, rather than too much, medication. If the patient does not get relief because of inadequate medication, he is likely to set up a continuous cry for more and more drugs, which will eventually lead to dependence. Medication should be prescribed in an appropriate manner, in times and amounts that meet the patient's needs for comfort on a continuing basis. Most patients can tolerate a moderate amount of pain as long as they are not forced to endure additional peaks that are not relieved.

The human desire to survive, to prolong life, is strong. The professional worker has no right to decide for the patient the course by which he should live out his remaining days. The spark of hope that he may need, even though in reality there is no hope, should not be destroyed. One patient revealed her mixture of reality and hope by saying, "You know, I always thought that if anyone told me I had cancer I'd kill myself. Now that I know, I see I really want to live after all, and hope that with the new drugs, I'll be able to." Another patient stated, "I had a feeling that I had a fatal disease, but it took me weeks to get used to the idea. Even though it seemed like I was doing all right on the surface, underneath I couldn't believe it. Now I think I should plan ahead anyway. After all, you never know."

If the physician has not worked through his own feelings regarding death and dying, and is unable to relate the truth to the patient, he may lose the patient's trust. This puts the nurse in the dilemma of being fearful lest she let something slip out in the course of conversation; it is still up to the physician to tell the patient his diagnosis.

The dying patient may well feel neglected and uncared for, as it seems that he must wait for everything—for the doctor to visit, for his family to come, for the nurse to respond to his buzzer, for the meal tray to be removed. Even the patient who isn't told his prognosis senses it and finds out the truth sooner or later. He picks up clues from the family, friends, or hospital workers. He is sensitive to false reassurance and gaiety. Some patients become very dependent and angry about being dependent. Consequently, they become hostile toward others.

A terminally ill patient feels deeply wounded. He does not want to be deserted. At times he feels rejected. He fears pain, or becoming ugly, unwanted, and unloved. He does not want to be considered repulsive and be avoided by others. He needs human contacts more than ever. To be alone during the long hours of his final journey is intolerable. He appreciates genuine gestures of warmth, sincerity, and closeness, even having someone just sit silently, sharing the moment by holding his hand. He may become obnoxious and angry and lash out with unjust and irrational remarks for no apparent reason. Especially at such times, he needs to be understood and befriended with compassion. He needs the chance to talk about his feelings and worries, and he also needs reassurance that his pain will be controlled.

Some patients refrain from speaking openly about their situation. Because of the imminence of death, patients often solve problems and difficulties that ordinarily would require a great deal of concentrated therapy. Whether or not he has been told his diagnosis, the patient knows that he is very sick. He will usually welcome the chance to tell you what he thinks he has, if he is asked. He may cry uncontrollably. Feelings of pain and discomfort are shared readily. Death may be mentioned in symbolic language, using disguised terms. The word "death" does not have to be used in answering questions or talking about deep concerns. Many times irrational fears and guilt associated with death can be alleviated and anxiety reduced by talking about the patient's feelings.

The patient's family may respond to his poor prognosis with anger. As he moves into the acceptance stage, they must be helped to know that he is accepting his dying and is gradually drifting away from them all. They need to be reassured that their behavior is not the cause of his speaking less frequently and dozing in their presence.

Patients who are terminally ill vary in their ability to reach the stage of preparation that leads to acceptance of death. The patient needs to set his own pace, and at intervals slides backward to a previous level. Staff should recognize the patient's undeniable right to ventilate his feelings and to employ other defense mechanisms as buffers in order to live as comfortably as he can for as long as he can.

Although terminally ill patients commonly react with anxiety and depression, there are other reactions which can occur in the face of death. One patient, when told that she had a fatal illness, became extremely promiscuous. She had multiple love affairs, attempting to induce men to impregnate her. Her drive to have a child was her way of denying and dealing with the prospect of her death. On the other hand, a fifty-two-year-old man demonstrated a heightened need to be close to his wife, to be held, fondled, touched, and caressed by her. The patient and his wife held fast to each other, markedly diminishing his sense of isolation and fear of abandonment.

In metastatic illness, the type of cancer and the treatment a patient receives may cause emotional problems, along with physical difficulties. For instance, a woman with metastatic breast cancer stated that the side effects of drug therapy, such as vomiting, constant nausea, and severe hair loss, were preventing her from enjoying what little time she had left. Another patient, with a permanent colostomy, felt disgust and humiliation. He was constantly concerned with the possibility of odors and with the change in his body image. He withdrew from his wife and family, claiming he was no longer the man that he thought he should be. His psychological impairment far exceeded the impairment created by his colostomy.

At times, it appears that some staff members have more difficulty with their own feelings about death and dying than the patient does with his. Evidence of this includes the worker's dislike for caring for the patient; inability to keep up ordinary conversation because of the worker's own discomfort; and anger at the patient's use of his defense mechanisms. At staff conferences about the dying, the following statements have been heard:

"Well, it's not the way I would want it, if I were the patient."

"I just don't know what to say to him. It's sad, and I'm afraid to talk about anything gay or happy because I feel like a phony."

"I want to reassure her that everything will be all right, but how can I?"

"I wish I could act blasé. I really do not want to talk about what is happening now."

"She pretends to be happy, as if she had all the time in the world. I wonder if I should go along with the act."

"What can one really do anyhow? You might as well care for someone where there will be positive results."

It is not uncommon for health workers to lose hope in the face of a patient's extensive treatment and to withdraw in an effort to protect themselves from the idea that they are adding to a patient's torture. Staff members may question additional treatments that do not reverse the disease process immediately or that cause additional pain. Often the health workers voice anger at the physician, projecting and displacing onto him their own sense of inadequacy.

It may be difficult for health care providers to realize that most patients will endure discomfort and hardship if there is even the slimmest chance that life can be extended or the illness halted, if only for a short time. The staff can be assisted to view their own negative reactions to ongoing treatments as part of their sense of impotence when the patient continues to deteriorate or dies. They need to be helped to tolerate the situation, rather than act out their anger by sabotaging the patient's treatment. By accepting what is happening they can help the patient cope with unpleasant or painful treatments that may bring the gift of a longer life.

Of course, there are times when, despite medication, treatment, and expert medical and nursing care, the inevitable must be accepted, and the health worker then recognizes his inability to "save" the patient. Often, his frustration is painful. His ability to cope with his sense of failure is lessened, thereby evoking a sense of impotence that results in feelings of extreme uselessness and hopelessness, causing him to withdraw from the patient long before death. This premature termination of the relationship cheats the patient of an important source of support as he nears death.

THE APPROACH TO THE TERMINALLY ILL PATIENT

Whenever possible, the staff member who feels most at ease with the patient and his family should be selected to work with the dying patient. This will make it easier for both patient and family to ventilate their feelings.

Make the patient comfortable. Do what you can to preserve his feelings of usefulness by encouraging him to perform whatever tasks he is able to carry out in connection with his care. Do not force him to talk if he doesn't want to, but be alert to signs that indicate his desire to talk and then provide opportunities for him to do so. Do not point out inconsistencies or contradictions when the patient talks. Recognize his need to deal with fear by confronting it at times and avoiding it at other times. Remember, the patient's defenses are allowing him to collect himself, so do not destroy them. Help him to resolve unfinished business or plans if he asks for this kind of assistance.

Accept the patient's anger. Do not react in such a way as to increase his sense of loneliness or to make him feel humiliated or guilty for having feelings of anger.

Offer yourself as a willing listener. Share his grief verbally or nonverbally. Let the patient know you understand the seriousness of his situation. Say, "This must be a difficult time for you." Do not avoid him. He interprets avoidance as a rejection of himself, not as your inability to deal with death.

Do not abandon the patient. Even when there is no possibility of a remission of his disease, approach him frequently, if only briefly. Never dampen his hopefulness. Respond with concern for his problems, no matter how trivial they may appear. Say, "This seems important to you. Let's see if we can settle it together."

Respect the patient's individuality and protect his right to die with dignity.

Suggested Readings

GENERAL BOOKS

Burton, Genevieve. *Personal, Impersonal, and Interpersonal Relations.* 3rd ed. New York: Springer Publishing Company, 1970.

Caplan, Gerald. *Concepts of Mental Health and Consultation.* Washington, D.C.: United States Department of Health, Education and Welfare, 1959.

Caplan, Gerald. *Principles of Preventive Psychiatry.* New York: Basic Books, 1964.

Davitz, Lois J. *Interpersonal Processes in Nursing—Case Histories.* New York: Springer Publishing Company, 1970.

Garrett, Annette. *Interviewing.* New York: Family Service Association of America, 1942.

Hofling, Charles K., M. Leininger, and E. Bregg. *Basic Psychiatric Concepts in Nursing.* 2nd ed. Philadelphia: J. B. Lippincott, 1967.

Kolb, Lawrence C. *Noyes' Modern Clinical Psychiatry.* 7th ed. Philadelphia: W. B. Saunders, 1968.

MacKinnon, Roger A., and Robert Mickels. *The Psychiatric Interview in Clinical Practice.* Philadelphia: W. B. Saunders, 1971.

Mathis, James L., C. M. Pierce, and V. Pishkin. *Basic Psychiatry: A Primer of Concepts and Terminology.* New York: Appleton-Century-Crofts, 1968.

Peplau, Hildegarde. *Interpersonal Relations in Nursing.* New York: G. P. Putnam's Sons, 1952.

Schwartz, M. S., and E. L. Shockley. *The Nurse and the Mental Patient.* New York: John Wiley, 1956.

Sullivan, Harry Stack. *The Psychiatric Interview.* New York: W. W. Norton, 1954.

Travelbee, Joyce. *Interpersonal Aspects of Nursing.* 2nd ed. Philadelphia: F. A. Davis, 1971.

Ujhely, Gertrud. *The Nurse and Her Problem Patients.* New York: Springer Publishing Company, 1963.

Ujhely, Gertrud. *Determinants of the Nurse-Patient Relationship.* New York: Springer Publishing Company, 1968.

LOOKING AT THE PATIENT

Bermosk, Loretta S. "Interviewing: A Key to Therapeutic Communication in Nursing," *Nursing Clinics of North America* (June, 1966).

Cummings, Jonathan W. "The Pressures and How Patients Respond," *American Journal of Nursing* 70:70–76 (January, 1970).

Dixson, Barbara K. "Intervening When the Patient Is Delusional," *Journal of Psychiatric Nursing and Mental Health Services* 9:25–31 (January-February, 1969).

Finestone, Albert J. "Medical Aspects of the Psychiatric Consultation," *Medical Times* 97:197–207 (August, 1969).

Foy, Audrey L. "Dreams of Patients and Staff," *American Journal of Nursing* 70:80–81 (January, 1970).

Rapport, Lydia. "The State of Crisis: Some Theoretical Considerations," *Social Service Review* 36:211–217 (February, 1962).

Scarf, Maggie. "Normality Is a Square Circle or a Four-Sided Triangle," *New York Times Magazine,* October 3, 1971, pp. 16, 17, 40, 41, 43–45, 48, 50.

LOOKING AT THE HEALTH WORKER

Deutsch, Helene. *The Psychology of Women.* 2 vols. New York: Grune and Stratton, 1945.

Foy, Audrey L. "Dreams of Patients and Staff," *American Journal of Nursing* 70:80–81 (January, 1970).

Nordmark, Madelyn T., and Anne W. Rohweder. *Scientific Foundations of Nursing.* 2nd ed. Philadelphia: J. B. Lippincott, 1967, pp. 259–335.

THE USE OF THE INTERVIEW

Bermosk, Loretta S. "Interviewing: A Key to Therapeutic Communication in Nursing," *Nursing Clinics of North America* (June, 1966).

Cummings, Jonathan W. "The Pressures and How Patients Respond," *American Journal of Nursing* 70:70–76 (January, 1970).

Davitz, Lois J. *The Psychiatric Patient–Case Histories.* Springer Publishing Company, 1971.

Dixson, Barbara K. "Intervening When the Patient Is Delusional," *Journal of Psychiatric Nursing and Mental Health Services* 9:25–31 (January-February, 1969).

Finestone, Albert J. "Medical Aspects of the Psychiatric Consultation," *Medical Times* 97:197–207 (August, 1969).

RESPECTING CONFIDENTIALITY

Bermosk, Loretta S. "Interviewing: A Key to Therapeutic Communication in Nursing," *Nursing Clinics of North America* (June, 1966).

THE HEALTH WORKER IN THE COMMUNITY

Fagin, C. M. *Family-Centered Nursing in Community Psychiatry.* Philadelphia: F. A. Davis, 1970.

Lewis, E. P., and M. H. Browning, eds. *The Nurse in Community Mental Health.* New York: The American Journal of Nursing Company, 1972.

CRISIS INTERVENTION

Augilera, D. C., and J. M. Messick. *Crisis Intervention.* St. Louis: C. V. Mosby Company, 1974.

Cummings, Jonathan W. "The Pressures and How Patients Respond," *American Journal of Nursing* 70:70–76 (January, 1970).

LeMasters, E. E. "Parenthood as Crisis," *Marriage and Family Living* 19: 352–372 (April, 1957).

Parad, Howard, ed. *Crisis Intervention: Selected Readings.* New York: Family Service Association of America, 1965.

Rapport, Lydia. "The State of Crisis: Some Theoretical Considerations," *Social Service Review* 36:211–217 (February, 1962).

THE ANXIOUS PATIENT

Cummings, Jonathan W. "The Pressures and How Patients Respond," *American Journal of Nursing* 70:70–76 (January, 1970).

THE DEPRESSED PATIENT

Cammer, Leonard. *Up from Depression.* New York: Simon and Schuster, 1969.

Enelow, Allen J., ed. *Depression in Medical Practice.* West Point, Pa: Merck, Sharp & Dohme, 1970.

Schneidman, Edwin S., and Larry H. Dizmang. "How the Family Physician Can Prevent Suicide," *The Physician's Panorama* 5:4–9 (June, 1967).

THE HELPLESS PATIENT

Mayfield, Betty, and Barr Doyce. "Ward Environment and the Severely Regressed Patient," *Journal of Psychiatric Nursing and Mental Health Services* 10:24–26 (May-June, 1972).

THE HALLUCINATING PATIENT

Grosicki, Jeanette P., and Marguerite Harmonson. "Nursing Action Guide: Hallucinations," *Journal of Psychiatric Nursing and Mental Health Services* 7:133–135 (May-June, 1969).

Lidz, Theodore, Stephen Fleck, and Alice R. Cornelison. *Schizophrenia and the Family.* New York: International Universities Press, 1967.

THE HOSTILE PATIENT

Rosenfeld, Ethel M. "Intervening in Hostile Behavior Through Dyadic and/or Group Intervention," *Journal of Psychiatric Nursing and Mental Health Services* 7:251-254 (November-December, 1969).

THE OBSESSIVE-COMPULSIVE PATIENT

Hadley, Alice A. H. "What is an Obsessive-Compulsive Neurosis?" in *Some Clinical Approaches to Psychiatric Nursing,* ed. Shirley F. Burd and Margaret A. Marshall. New York: Macmillan Company, 1963, pp. 81-86.

THE PATIENT WITH A PSYCHIATRIC EMERGENCY

Dixson, Barbara K. "Intervening When the Patient Is Delusional," *Journal of Psychiatric Nursing and Mental Health Services* 9:25-31 (January-February, 1969).

Fromm-Reichmann, Frieda. *Principles of Intensive Psychotherapy.* Chicago: University of Chicago Press, 1950.

Lidz, Theodore, Stephen Fleck, and Alice R. Cornelison. *Schizophrenia and the Family.* New York: International Universities Press, 1967.

Schneidman, Edwin S., and Larry H. Dizmang. "How the Family Physician Can Prevent Suicide," *The Physician's Panorama* 5:4-9 (June, 1967).

Singer, Erwin. *Key Concepts in Psychotherapy.* 2nd ed. New York: Basic Books, 1970.

THE PATIENT RECEIVING ELECTROSTIMULATIVE TREATMENT

Miller, Edgar. "Psychological Theories of ECT: A Review," *International Journal of Psychiatry* 5:154-163 (February, 1968).

264 *Suggested Readings*

THE DRUG OR ALCOHOL DEPENDENT PATIENT

Childress, Gwendolyn. "The Role of the Nurse with the Drug Abuser and
Addict," *Journal of Psychiatric Nursing and Mental Health Services*
8:21–26 (March-April, 1970).
Dole, P. Vincent. "Narcotic Addiction, Physical Dependence and Relapse,"
The New England Journal of Medicine 286:988–992 (May 4, 1972).
Ehrhardt, Helmut E. "Drug Dependence: Actual Problems of Significance,
Spreading, Treatment and Control," *Journal of Psychiatric Nursing
Gershon, Samuel, and Burton Angrist. "Drug-Induced Psychoses: I,"
Hospital Practice (June, 1967), pp. 36–39.
Klee, Gerald D. "Drugs and American Youth," *Medical Times* 97:165–171
(August, 1969).
Kolansky, Harold, and William T. Moore. "Effects of Marihuana on
Adolescents and Young Adults," *Journal of Psychiatric Nursing and
Mental Health Services* 9:9–16 (November-December, 1971).
Murray, Alice. "Alcohol: Affliction of 110,000 on L.I.," *The New York
Times,* January 23, 1972, p. 1.
Stuart, R. B. *Behavioral Self-Management.* New York: Brunner/Mazel,
1977.

THE ACUTELY SUICIDAL PATIENT

Floyd, G. J. "Nursing Management of the Suicidal Patient," *Journal of
Psychiatric Nursing and Mental Health Services* 13:23–26 (March-
April, 1975).
Kastenbaum, Robert. *The Psychology of Death.* New York: Springer
Publishing Company, 1972.
Leonard, C. V. "Treating the Suicidal Patient: A Communication Ap-
13:19–22 (March-April, 1975).

THE PATIENT WITH SEXUAL PROBLEMS

Abbott, Marcia A. "Resuming Sexual Activity After Myocardial Infarc-

Browning, M. H., and E. P. Lewis, eds. *Human Sexuality: Nursing Implications.* New York: The American Journal of Nursing Company, 1973.

Burgess, A. W., A. N. Groth, L. L. Holmstrom, and S. M. Sgroi. *Sexual Assault of Children and Adolescents.* Lexington, Mass.: Lexington Books, 1978.

Cassem, Ned H., and T. P. Hackett. "Psychological Aspects of Myocardial Infarction," *The Medical Clinics of North America* 61:711-721 (July, 1977).

Churchill, W. *Homosexual Behavior Among Males.* Englewood Cliffs, N.J.: Prentice-Hall, 1971.

Gadpaille, W. J. *The Cycles of Sex.* New York: Scribner's, 1975.

Greggs, Winona. "Sex and the Elderly," *American Journal of Nursing* 78: 1352-1354 (August, 1978).

Grimm, E. R. "Women's Attitudes and Reactions to Childbearing," in *Modern Woman: Her Psychology and Sexuality,* ed. G. D. Goldman and D. S. Nilman. Springfield, Ill.: Charles C Thomas, 1969, pp. 129-163.

Kaplan, H. S. *The New Sex Therapy.* New York: Brunner-Mazel, 1974.

Katchadourian, H. A., and D. T. Lunde. *Fundamentals of Human Sexuality.* New York: Holt, Rinehart and Winston, 1972.

Masters, W. H., and V. E. Johnson. *The Pleasure Bond.* Boston: Little, Brown, 1974.

Reuben, D. R. *Everything You Always Wanted to Know About Sex.* New York: David McKay Company, 1970.

Sadock, B. J., H. I. Kaplan, and A. M. Freedman, eds. *The Sexual Experience.* Baltimore: Williams and Wilkins, 1976.

THE PATIENT WITH SOMATIC COMPLAINTS

Arieti, S., ed. *American Handbook of Psychiatry.* Vol. 4. New York: Basic Books, 1975, pp. 477-922.

THE PATIENT WITH ANOREXIA NERVOSA

Alvarez, W. C. "Nervous Loss of Appetite," *Newsday.* July 21, 1972, p. 16A.

Barcai, A. "Family Therapy in the Treatment of Anorexia Nervosa," *American Journal of Psychiatry* 3:286-290 (1971).

Bruch, H. "Family Background in Eating Disorders," in *The Child in his Family*. ed. E. J. Anthony and C. Koupernik. New York: John Wiley, 1970.

Dikowitz, S. "Anorexia Nervosa," *Journal of Psychiatric Nursing and Mental Health Services* 14:28-37 (October, 1976).

King, D. A. "Anorexic Behavior: A Nursing Problem," *Journal of Psychiatric Nursing and Mental Health Services* 9:11-17 (May-June, 1971).

Lipkin, G. B. *Parent-Child Nursing: Psychosocial Aspects*. St. Louis: C. V. Mosby Company, 1978, p. 208-209.

Palazzoli, M. S. *Self-Starvation*. New York: Jason Aronson, 1978.

Schlemmer, K., and P. Barnett. "Management of Manipulative Behavior of Anorexia Nervosa Patients," *Journal of Psychiatric Nursing and Mental Health Services* 15:35-41 (November, 1977).

THE DIABETIC PATIENT

Arnold, Helen M. "Elderly Diabetic Amputees," *American Journal of Nursing* 69:2646-2649 (December, 1969).

Brunner, Lillian Sholtis, L. Emerson, Jr., and Ferguson Suddarth. *Textbook of Medical-Surgical Nursing*. Philadelphia: J. B. Lippincott, 1964, pp. 507-567, 309-347, 826-838.

Nordmark, Madelyn T., and Anne W. Rohweder. *Scientific Foundations of Nursing*. 2nd ed. Philadelphia: J. B. Lippincott, 1967, pp. 259-335.

Stuart, Sarah. "Day-to-Day Living with Diabetes," *American Journal of Nursing* 71:1548-1550 (August, 1971).

THE PATIENT WITH A MASTECTOMY

Quint, Jeanne C. "The Impact of Mastectomy," *American Journal of Nursing* 63:89-92 (November, 1963).

THE PATIENT WITH CORONARY HEART DISEASE

Andreoli, K., V. Hunn, D. P. Zipes, and A. G. Wallace. *Comprehensive Cardiac Care: A Handbook for Nurses and Other Paramedical Personnel.* St. Louis: C. V. Mosby Company, 1968.

Brunner, Lillian Sholtis, L. Emerson, Jr., and Ferguson Suddarth. *Textbook of Medical-Surgical Nursing.* Philadelphia: J. B. Lippincott, 1964, pp. 507-567, 309-347, 826-838.

Cassem, N. H., and Thomas P. Hackett. "Psychiatric Consultation in a Coronary Care Unit," *Annals of Internal Medicine* 75:9-14 (July, 1971).

Crews, Judy. "Nurse-Managed Cardiac Clinics," *Cardio-Vascular Nursing* 8:15-18 (July-August, 1972).

Gentry, W. O., and R. B. Williams, eds. *Psychological Aspects of Myocardial Infarction and Coronary Care.* St. Louis: C. V. Mosby Company, 1975.

Harris, Raymond, R. M. Kohn, B. Kutner, and F. A. Whitehouse. "Rehabilitation of the Cardiac Patient," *New York State Journal of Medicine* 70:511-513 (February 15, 1970).

Levine, Herbert. "What the Coronary Care Unit Meant to Me," *Medical Times* 98:124-131 (September, 1970).

Nickel, Vernon L. "Rehabilitation to Improve Function in Stroke Patients," *Current Concepts of Cerebrovascular Disease* 6:7-10 (March-April, 1971).

Nordmark, Madelyn T., and Anne W. Rohweder. *Scientific Foundations of Nursing.* 2nd ed. Philadelphia: J. B. Lippincott, 1967, pp. 259-335.

Perlman, Lawrence V., S. Fergusen, K. Bergum, L. Isenberg, and J. F. Hammarstein. "Precipitation of Congestive Heart Failure: Social and Emotional Factors," *Annals of Internal Medicine* 75:1-7 (July, 1971).

Steincrohn, Peter J. *Your Heart Is Stronger than You Think.* New York: Cowles Book Company, 1970.

Twerski, Abraham. "Psychological Considerations on the Coronary Care Unit," *Cardio-Vascular Nursing* 7:65-68 (March-April, 1971).

Whitehouse, Frederick A. "Advising the Patient," *Cardiac Rehabilitation* 2:23-27 (Summer, 1971).

THE PATIENT UNDERGOING RENAL DIALYSIS OR TRANSPLANT

Bois, Marna S., B. Barfield, E. Taylor, and C. Ross. "The Patient with a Kidney Transplant," *American Journal of Nursing* 68:1238-1239, 1242-1247 (June, 1968).

Brunner, Lillian Sholtis, L. Emerson, Jr., and Ferguson Suddarth. *Textbook of Medical-Surgical Nursing.* Philadelphia: J. B. Lippincott, 1964, pp. 507-567, 309-347, 826-838.

Hickman, B. W. "All About Sex . . . Despite Dialysis," *American Journal of Nursing* 77:606-607 (April, 1977).

Kobrzycki, P. "Renal Transplant Complications," *American Journal of Nursing* 77:641-643 (April, 1977).

Martin, Alfred J. "Renal Transplantation: Surgical Technique and Complications," *American Journal of Nursing* 68:1240-1241 (June, 1968).

Nordmark, Madelyn T., and Anne W. Rohweder. *Scientific Foundations of Nursing.* 2nd ed. Philadelphia: J. B. Lippincott, 1967, pp. 259-335.

Schlotter, Lowanna. "What Do You Teach the Dialysis Patient," *American Journal of Nursing* 70:82-83 (January, 1970).

THE PEDIATRIC PATIENT

Ailitt, Ada Hart. *Psychology of Infancy and Early Childhood.* 3rd ed. New York: McGraw-Hill, 1946.

Bergmann, Thesi, in collaboration with Anna Freud. *Children in the Hospital.* New York: International Universities Press, 1965.

Brody, Jane E. "Adults Are Advised to be Honest with a Dying Child," *The New York Times,* January 23, 1972, p. 9.

Burgert, Omer E. "Emotional Impact of Childhood Acute Leukemia," *Mayo Clinic Proceedings* 47:273-277 (April, 1972).

Chess, S., and M. Hassibi. *Principles and Practice of Child Psychiatry.* New York: Plenum Press, 1978.

Freud, Anna. *Normality and Pathology in Childhood.* New York: International Universities Press, 1965.

Mahler, M. S., F. Pine, and A. Bergman. *The Psychological Birth of the Human Infant.* New York: Basic Books, 1975.

Martin, Alfred J. "Renal Transplantation: Surgical Technique and Complications," *American Journal of Nursing* 68:1240–1241 (June, 1968).

Smith, Margo. "Ego Support for the Child Patient," *American Journal of Nursing* 63:90–95 (October, 1963).

Sperling, Melitta. *The Major Neuroses and Behavior Disorders in Children.* New York: Jason Aronson, 1974.

Sperling, Melitta. *Psychosomatic Disorders in Childhood.* New York: Jason Aronson, 1978.

THE ADOLESCENT PATIENT

Alvarez, Walter C. "Nervous Loss of Appetite," *Newsday,* July 21, 1972, p. 16A.

Blum, Sam. "Marijuana Clouds the Generation Gap," *The New York Times Magazine,* August 23, 1970, pp. 28, 48, 55, 58.

Jacobs, J. *Adolescent Suicide.* New York: Wiley-Interscience, 1971.

Jurgensen, Kathleen. "Limit Setting for Hospitalized Adolescent Psychiatric Patients," *Perspectives in Psychiatric Care* 9:173–183 (July-August, 1971).

Kagan, J. R. Coles. *Twelve to Sixteen: Early Adolescence.* New York: W. W. Norton, 1972.

King, Dorothy A. "Anorexic Behavior: A Nursing Problem," *Journal of Psychiatric Nursing and Mental Health Services* 9:11–17 (May-June, 1971).

Klee, Gerald D. "Drugs and American Youth," *Medical Times* 97:165–171 (August, 1969).

Kolansky, Harold, and William T. Moore. "Effects of Marihuana on Adolescents and Young Adults," *Journal of Psychiatric Nursing and Mental Health Services* 9:9–16 (November-December, 1971).

Miller, D. *Adolescence.* New York: Jason Aronson, 1974.

THE PATIENT WITH A POSTPARTUM PSYCHOSIS

Gordon, R. E., and K. K. Gordon. "Social Factors in the Prediction and Treatment of Emotional Disorders of Pregnancy," *American Journal of Obstetrics and Gynecology* 77:197-207 (May, 1959).

Grimm, Elaine R. "Women's Attitudes and Reactions to Childbearing," in *Modern Woman: Her Psychology and Sexuality,* ed. George D. Goldman and Donald S. Nilman. Springfield, Ill.: Charles C Thomas, 1969, pp. 129-163.

Hemilton, J. A. *Postpartum Psychiatric Problems.* St. Louis: C. V. Mosby, 1962.

LeMasters, E. E. "Parenthood as Crisis," *Marriage and Family Living* 19:352-372 (April, 1957).

Lipkin, G. B. *Antepartal Anticipatory Guidance Conferences and Postpartum Blues.* Unpublished thesis, Adelphi University, Garden City, N.Y.

Robin, A. A. "The Psychological Changes of Normal Parturition," *Psychiatric Quarterly* 36:129-249 (January, 1962).

Wenner, N. K., et al. "Emotional Problems in Pregnancy," *Psychiatry* 32:389-410 (November, 1969).

Yalom, I. D., et al. "Postpartum Blues Syndrome," *Archives of General Psychiatry* 18:16-27 (January, 1968).

THE AGED PATIENT

Burnside, I. M. *Psychosocial Nursing Care of the Aged.* New York: McGraw-Hill, 1973.

Burnside, I. M. "Recognizing and Reducing Emotional Problems in the Aged," *Nursing '77* 7:56-59 (March, 1977).

Kahana, Ralph J. "Common Psychiatric Problems in Aged Patients Admitted to the General Hospital," *Hospital Medicine* 7:104-109 (June, 1967).

THE TERMINALLY ILL PATIENT

Kastenbaum, Robert. *The Psychology of Death.* New York: Springer
Publishing Company, 1972.
Krant, M. J. *Dying and Dignity.* Springfield, Ill.: Charles C Thomas, 1974.
Kübler-Ross, E. *Death–The Final Stage of Growth.* Englewood Cliffs,
N.J.: Prentice-Hall, 1975.
Ostheimer, N. C., and J. M. Ostheimer, eds. *Life or Death–Who Controls.*
New York: Springer Publishing Company, 1976.
Rosenbaum, E. H. *Living With Cancer.* New York: Praeger Publishers,
1975.

Index